Praise for
Loving Someone
with Borderline Personality Disorder

"This hopeful yet realistic book is an indispensable tool for managing relationships with persons who have borderline personality disorder. Research based, clearly written, and practical, this guide to a complex disorder is highly recommended."
—*Library Journal*

"More than many other disorders, BPD affects relationships. This book offers families and friends invaluable skills for helping both their loved one and themselves. Dr. Manning has done a beautiful job. A 'must read.'"
—*Perry D. Hoffman, PhD, President, National Education Alliance for Borderline Personality Disorder*

"This book opened my eyes to BPD! I wanted to understand what my friend was going through and help as much as possible. I was amazed to find that the techniques in the book really did help me respond differently during one of her episodes, when I normally would have just gotten angry. Our communication (and my feelings toward her) have truly benefited."
—*R. P., South Carolina*

"Dr. Manning's compassion, understanding, and nonjudgmental approach resonate on every page of this readable, helpful book. She eloquently describes the challenges of caring for someone with BPD and provides numerous step-by-step strategies for dealing with common problems."
—*Michaela Swales, PhD, School of Psychology, Bangor University, United Kingdom*

"The title says it all! Dr. Manning explains what she has learned about the true nature of BPD from the experts themselves—those who have the disorder. She shows family and friends how our instinctive responses to the crises associated with BPD are frequently ineffective or even harmful, and illuminates what we can do differently, providing practical, incisive, step-by-step guidance. The book helps readers understand their complicated relationship with a person with severe emotion dysregulation. It provides valuable tools for dealing with self-harm, suicidality, and hospitalization decisions. Of crucial importance, Dr. Manning clearly affirms that BPD—and the pain experienced by those who suffer—is *real*. We highly recommend this book."
—*Jim and Diane Hall, parents of an adult child with BPD and Family Educators for the National Alliance on Mental Illness and the National Education Alliance for Borderline Personality Disorder*

"Try out the recommendations this book gives you. You will be surprised by how much better your relationships become."
—*from the Foreword by Marsha M. Linehan, PhD, Director, Behavioral Research and Training Clinics, University of Washington*

Loving Someone
with Borderline Personality Disorder

Loving Someone

with Borderline Personality Disorder

How to Keep Out-of-Control Emotions
from Destroying Your Relationship

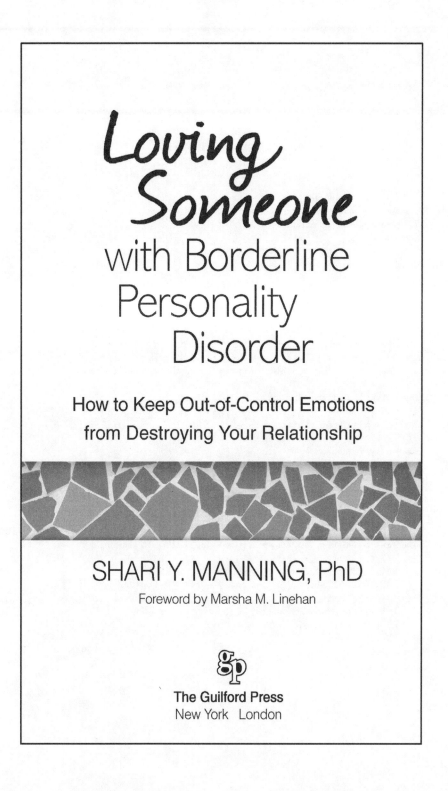

SHARI Y. MANNING, PhD

Foreword by Marsha M. Linehan

The Guilford Press

New York   London

The information in this volume is not intended as a substitute for consultation with healthcare professionals. Each individual's health concerns should be evaluated by a qualified professional.

Printed in the United States of America

This book is printed on acid-free paper.

Last digit is print number: 9   8   7

Library of Congress Cataloging-in-Publication Data

Manning, Shari Y.

    Loving someone with borderline personality disorder : how to keep out-of-control emotions from destroying your relationship / by Shari Y. Manning.
        p.   cm.
    Includes bibliographical references and index.
    ISBN 978-1-59385-607-6 (pbk. : alk. paper) — ISBN 978-1-60918-195-6 (hardcover : alk. paper)
    1. Borderline personality disorder.   2. Interpersonal relations.   I. Title.
    RC569.5.B67M356 2011
    158.2087′4—dc22

                                          2011007931

*For Elizabeth Younis Bush (Mama),
who has always been exactly
the mother I needed*

Contents

*P*ART I

Understanding Your Loved One and Your Relationship

$\mathcal{P}$ART II

The Many Faces of Borderline Personality Disorder

$\mathcal{P}$ART III

Dealing with Crisis and Getting Help

Foreword

Borderline personality disorder (BPD) is one of the most stigmatized mental disorders. Popular books about BPD may make readers cringe and want to run away from anyone who meets the criteria for the disorder. Mental health professionals frequently refuse to accept into treatment people diagnosed with BPD. Even in routine medical settings, the diagnosis can be the "kiss of death" for receiving tender loving care.

I cannot count the number of phone calls we get at my research clinic from mothers and fathers, daughters and sons, brothers and sisters, husbands and wives, current and past lovers, and even coworkers of individuals who meet the criteria for BPD. The questions are usually twofold: (1) "How can we survive this person?" and (2) "How can we help this person we love?" A third set of questions sometimes arises: "Am I a bad person? Why can't I make him [or her] happy?" The basic message is "HELP ME!" Often these initial phone calls lead to in-person consultations. Sometimes multiple sessions are needed to provide any help at all.

At my clinic at the University of Washington, we offer a skills training group specifically for the family and friends of individuals who meet the criteria for BPD. The skills are the same ones taught to the individuals with BPD in our dialectical behavior therapy (DBT) treatment program. DBT skills (mindfulness, emotion regulation, crisis survival, reality acceptance, and interpersonal effectiveness) have been shown to reduce emotion dysregulation, anger, and impulsive behavior. But such a skills program can only reach so many people. Attending it requires that those who want to help someone come into treatment themselves—a difficult thing to ask for or to do.

What if, instead of having to go to therapy to get help, you could find a good book that would tell you how to do it? This is such a book. It is written by an expert in treating BPD, an expert in DBT, and a person who has spent much of her life teaching others how to effectively treat and, yes, to love individuals with BPD. Shari Manning has worked with relatives for whom the central questions were "Should I leave or stay?" or "Should I send the person somewhere out of the house and away from me for therapy?" She knows what she is talking about.

Dr. Manning's first step is helping you understand the person with BPD. This understanding is, of course, central if you are to find your way back to loving the person with whom you are so often furious. She then introduces the DBT validation skills that are a central part of the strategies taught to therapists as well as a critical set of skills taught to clients and family members. *Validation* is communicating understanding to another person in a nonjudgmental fashion. It communicates that you take the person seriously and respect his or her point of view. It says to the other person that you see the wisdom in his or her behavior. Dr. Manning then takes the six levels of DBT validation and shows you how to make them your own, with many examples and explanations of how to use validation to improve your relationships.

What is wonderful about Part II of the book is that you will understand the behavior of the person you love far better than you ever have before. Even more important is Dr. Manning's ability to explain really painful behaviors in a way that reduces rather than increases judgmental reactions. Love requires acceptance.

In Part III, Dr. Manning provides guidelines for managing the most difficult set of problems: handling your own emotions and figuring out how to respond to a suicidal person who is close to you. These are two issues that even the most seasoned therapist finds difficult to manage. Here you get guidelines from an expert.

In sum, if you wish to preserve love and compassion and use skillful means, even when love, compassion, and skillful means seem impossible, this is the book for you. I believe you will find it helpful in improving your relationships with even those difficult people in your life who do not have BPD. Try out the recommendations this book gives you. You will be surprised by how much better your relationships become.

MARSHA M. LINEHAN, PhD
University of Washington, Seattle

Acknowledgments

When I was 16 years old, I decided that I wanted to work at the South Carolina State Hospital. I had been to the grounds to visit Paul Van Wyke, a family friend who was a psychologist at SCSH, and was fascinated by what I saw there. When I was 18, the movie *Ordinary People* was released, and I decided that I wanted to work with people who were suicidal. At 25, I was teaching school and studying for my master's degree. I discovered that the head cheerleader at the school was a "cutter" and I started working with her for my practicum. After she had an overdose that led to admission to a psychiatric facility, my supervisor, Carl Rak, PhD, told me that I was working with a young woman with borderline personality disorder (BPD), and he began educating me on BPD. Most of all, he began helping me develop compassion for people with BPD. By the end of that school year, I had my life plan: I wanted to work with severely suicidal people who had BPD.

In 1993, I was working in community mental health and studying for my doctorate. I was known as the clinician in the clinic who was always willing to work with people with BPD, but I wasn't effective. Luckily, Columbia Area Mental Health Center agreed that I wasn't effective and began to invest resources in finding a treatment for BPD. The next thing I knew, I was at Duke University beginning a 6-month course of study with Marsha Linehan, PhD, in an exciting new treatment for BPD called dialectical behavior therapy (DBT). Marsha and her work in DBT have defined my life, personally and professionally.

Those who practice DBT are compassionate and dedicated to understanding the experience of BPD but at the same time believe, unwaveringly, that the most compassionate thing we can do is help people with BPD to change.

Marsha has been a colleague, a mentor, a friend, and, along with my mother, the greatest influence in my life. There are not enough words to express my appreciation for her contribution to the field and to my life's work. In spite of having the busiest schedule I have ever known, Marsha has taken the time to talk through parts of this book with me. I can always count on her honest critiques and her guidance.

My colleagues at Behavioral Tech and Behavioral Tech Research (especially Cindy Beil, Kathy Satre, Linda Dimeff, and Sarah Schlossman) have had a part in the creation of this book. They talked through sections, they made sure I had weekends to write (sometimes locked in hotel rooms), and they encouraged me every step of the way. One Saturday at our annual behavior therapy conference, Helen Best spent hours talking to me about the book and all of my hopes for it and the fears that were keeping me from writing. It would never have gotten finished if Helen hadn't intervened.

Julie Skutch was my cheerleader. She would ask if I was writing and tell me that I needed to get the book finished, and she read the final draft. I counted on Julie to tell me if I was being judgmental or invalidating, and I knew she would do so.

I am blessed with friends who know how to support without putting on too much pressure. Ann Dwyer, Debbie Peagler, and Melissa Williams asked about my progress, encouraged me to keep going, and made me feel special. Thanks for boat rides and afternoons when I could take a little vacation.

If Marsha Linehan and DBT are the foundation of this book, Kitty Moore and Chris Benton of The Guilford Press are the framework. When I wanted to quit, they didn't let me. When work got overwhelming and I disappeared, they hunted me down and got me back to work. When so many things in my life were working against this book, they worked for it. We had these wonderful phone calls where Chris and Kitty would say, "How do you do this?" or "What do you think of this?" and we would talk for hours about everything I wanted to say. They became a big part of my life and I will miss our calls.

The clients and families in this book are all based on real people (although I've protected their privacy by changing names and identifying details and often by creating composites of several people). They had difficulties, but they had love and perseverance. What DBT taught me about how to conduct therapy, my patients and families taught me about the power of love to create a platform for change.

Finally, my husband, Jim Manning, has always believed in me. He started telling me years ago that this book was inside of me. He has given me time, missed days on the boat while I was locked up in my room writing, and never once complained. He is steadfast and has shown me how important it is to have someone who really is your biggest fan. If I hadn't had his love and support, this book would not have been written.

Loving Someone
with Borderline Personality Disorder

Introduction

"How could she do that to me—and herself—over and over?"

"Why would anyone act like that?"

"I don't know how much more I can take. But I've left before, and I keep coming back. What's wrong with *me*?"

"How can I possibly help him when I have no idea where to start?"

If you love someone with borderline personality disorder (BPD), you've probably asked all of these questions at some point or other, maybe repeatedly. Whether you're a spouse or partner, a parent, a sibling, or a close friend, having a relationship with someone who has this problem can be exhausting and exasperating. People with this disorder are impulsive and unpredictable. They may frighten the ones they love, and they're certainly destructive to themselves. They seem to be surrounded by chaos wherever they go and career from crisis to crisis, often taking their loved ones along for the ride.

So why are you reading this book? Why don't you just get out and be done with it?

Probably because people with BPD are also tremendously compassionate and caring. They love people and animals. They are usually smart and funny. Most of us see the potential in the people we love with BPD. We just know that they could be so wonderful *if* they could change some things in their lives.

This is why we stay when we may frequently believe we really should go. But in your case it may also be because you're tied to this person by blood, and you're not about to abandon your daughter or your brother. Or you still see plenty of evidence of the person you found so appealing when you made a conscious decision to enter this relationship, and that's the person you want to hold on to.

This book is intended to help you do that. I'm not going to tell you that in 10 easy steps you can make the person you love change in the ways that seem so clearly necessary to everyone around him or her. I'm not going to give you a few magic words that will make your next ultimatum stick, keep your phone from ringing off the hook at 3:00 A.M., or finally ensure that your loved one understands you have feelings too.

What I am going to do in this book is help you understand how BPD can make people who seem to have so much going for them behave in such bafflingly destructive and self-destructive ways. Your life can improve exponentially when you know what the internal experience of your loved one is like. Your compassionate understanding can lead you to effective new ways to interact that all by themselves may make it possible for you to stay in a relationship that has already taken so much of your energy and devotion. Using some fairly straightforward new ways to respond to your loved one that are provided in this book, you gain the power to change the outcome of historically painful and frustrating encounters. With time, these simple strategies just might help the person you love surmount some of the effects of BPD and leave you both free to enjoy the relationship you've always wanted to have.

Incidentally, this book assumes that the person in your life who has borderline personality disorder could be either male or female, so I've alternated between feminine and masculine pronouns throughout. You'll also find anecdotes and illustrations about both women and men in the book, because that reflects the reality of my professional experiences. (The anecdotes are based on real people, but all names and identifying details have been changed, and in fact most stories represent composites of people I have known.) Some people believe that borderline personality disorder is much more common among women than men, but the current data are unclear, and both research evidence and clinical observation tell me it's on the rise among men. New data show that 50% of those diagnosed with BPD are men.

I know that by the time you seek out this book, the demands of

BPD are likely to have worn you out. A lot of people who love someone with this condition end up feeling as if they have no control over
what happens to them, and this can be the most depleting feeling of all.
Please know that one of my primary goals is to help you ensure your own
well-being. You can't try to help your loved one change or fight to save
your relationship if you don't take care of yourself. Fortunately, you'll
find that the new ways of interacting described in this book can protect
you, even restoring your sense of who you are and what's important to
you. There's a lot you can do to make sure you don't end up the victim
of your loved one's illness. There's also a rational approach to knowing
whether you've reached the point where enough really is enough—one
that depends on knowing your own heart and mind rather than relying
on the influence of well-meaning others who insist you're being "manipulated" and "exploited."

The truth, as you'll learn in this book, is that your loved one is not
a terrible person, as much as he or she may have a pattern of some pretty
terrible behavior. It's not that your partner or family member *wants* to
create chaos or make anyone miserable. It's that your loved one *can't* do
the right thing, get along with others, or make the choices that seem
so plainly correct to everyone else—*because he or she doesn't know how*.
That may seem awfully hard to grasp. Doesn't everyone just have a feel
for what it takes to keep a job or a friend, how much is too much to ask of
those who care about us, and how to exercise a little self-control? Wasn't
your loved one born with the same instincts and the same opportunities
to learn how to navigate the world as the rest of us?

As difficult as it is to believe, the answer is no. People with BPD were
born with an invisible, innate difference that profoundly changed the
landscape for them when they were growing up. When you understand
this difference, their enigmatic behavior suddenly becomes remarkably
clear. You'll see what I mean starting in the first few chapters of this
book.

As I said, there's no set of foolproof steps to produce change in your
loved one, and your understanding isn't going to lead to total transfor-
mation. But as you'll see in the rest of the book, it can make a pretty
radical difference, one of much greater magnitude than understanding, say, why an alcoholic drinks or why someone you know can't be
in the same room with a spider. I'll show you how some straightforward
changes in the way you respond to your loved one can make your days

happier and even head off a lot of the crisis-generating behavior that keeps sapping your strength and weakening your resolve to stick by this person you care about so much.

The practical suggestions that you'll be reading about in this book are all based on the treatment that has proved most effective for people with BPD. It's called *dialectical behavior therapy* (DBT), and it was created by Marsha M. Linehan at the University of Washington. This therapy has been widely tested and shown to make tremendous headway toward giving people with the disorder skills that elude them and that the rest of us often take for granted. You can't—and should not—try to serve as your loved one's therapist, of course, but you can certainly benefit from the same principles that a qualified DBT therapist would use to help your loved one. Your loved one may have been diagnosed with this disorder or may have some of its symptoms, and maybe he or she is receiving treatment. You can use this book to help you in your relationship whether the person you love is in treatment or not. I strongly recommend, if your loved one is not receiving treatment, that DBT be considered. Toward the end of this book you'll find information on DBT and how it helps.

Meanwhile, take care of yourself by reading this book. I hope it will help you preserve a bond that is so important to you and lead the two of you to a happier future together.

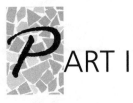

PART I

Understanding Your Loved One and Your Relationship

"Why Do I Feel So Lost in This Relationship?"

Someone I know recently fulfilled a life goal: he married a wonderful woman. About 2 months later, though, things began to change. The woman he had married asked him for a significant sum of money to start a business. He told her he didn't have that kind of money and was completely unprepared for the emotional reaction he got. She first became really angry and berated him for not loving her enough. She picked up a paperweight and threatened to throw it at him. Then she became despondent and said she didn't deserve to live. Finally, she drank a bottle of wine and burned herself several times on the arm with a cigarette.

That one evening became a turning point in their relationship. The wife quit her job. She vacillated between not speaking with my friend for hours and spending hours telling him what a bad person he was. She often drank two bottles of wine in an evening. She went into great detail about how worthless she was. My friend tried to get his wife help, but she mostly refused. After he had to leave the house several times because his wife was out of control, friends and family began to tell him to leave her. The problem with leaving his wife, however, was that she was not always despondent, drunk, and enraged. There were moments when my friend saw the woman he had fallen in love with, a woman who was smart, witty, caring, and exciting. He wanted to be with that woman.

Meanwhile, the psychiatrist who had seen his wife a couple of times told my friend that his wife met the criteria for borderline personality disorder (BPD). He was very discouraging. In fact he told him that there was no help for his wife and that he should just get out of the relationship before things got worse. My friend is still with his wife, but he's often exhausted and stressed out and seems less and less like the outgoing, optimistic person I've known.

*H*ow Borderline Behavior Can Make You Lose Your Balance

My friend, whose name is Brad, describes himself these days as feeling generally lost. A man with the enviable knack for knowing just the right thing to say or do in virtually any situation, he now says that everything he does with regard to his wife, whose name is Sadie, seems to be wrong. Brad no longer trusts his social instincts, and friends have started to notice that he often retreats into a corner at gatherings where he'd usually be at the epicenter. After the fateful conversation where he told his new wife that he couldn't give her thousands of dollars, he agonized all night over whether he was in fact being stingy and had underestimated what he could afford to do without. It was only the first of many sleepless nights spent second-guessing simple decisions that seemed so benign at the time but got such an accusatory reaction from Sadie. Surely he must have done something offensive if his wife was that upset, he told himself. So he would rehash the incident again and again, looking for an explanation but never able to find a credible middle ground between the idea that he was the terrible person Sadie had called him and the idea that *she* was. He wasn't quite sure who he was anymore, and he certainly didn't know who Sadie was.

> When everything you do seems to be wrong, you can quickly lose your self-confidence.

Brad's confusion was compounded by the fact that sometimes Sadie was everything he'd ever wanted in a wife. Once, after hearing the discouragement in his voice when she called him at work and asked how his day was going, she surprised him by having a candlelit dinner all ready when he got home and a DVD of an obscure old movie he'd mentioned months ago that he'd always wanted to see. When his mother was recovering from surgery and he was caught up in the busiest time of year at his job, Sadie had doted on his mother so Brad didn't have to worry about how she was managing on her own. Two of his friends kept asking him when they could all get together for dinner again because the last time they'd gone out Sadie had had everyone in convulsions as she told one hilarious story after the next. Sometimes Brad felt like he was living with two different women, and he wondered whether he was simply losing his mind.

Of course he wasn't. The fact is that there are so many reasons we love people with BPD. Most are kind and generous of spirit. One time I had surgery, and after returning to run a group with eight women who had BPD diagnoses, I casually remarked that my husband was not doing such a good job of cooking for me while I was recovering. The next week, every woman in the group brought me some kind of casserole.

When someone acts so caring, you can easily question whether your anger at the aggressive, frightening behavior that you see at other times is justifiable, as Brad did. Maybe, you might think, you're not a very good or worthy judge of human character at all. Or you get overinvolved. In training therapists, I have often found that therapists who treat BPD can lose their way simply because their clients are so kind and such brilliant listeners that the therapists feel like the clients are taking care of them instead of the other way around. Then they feel an irresistible urge to repay the clients in kind and end up extending themselves in inappropriate ways. For example, I knew of a therapist at one point who loaned a great deal of money to a client. I once met another one who called her client when she, the therapist, was in emotional distress. A third I know of ended up adopting the daughter of a client. All of these behaviors are considered questionable or unethical in our profession, and I know the therapists did not set out to be unethical. Somehow the behaviors typical of someone with BPD made them lose their way.

Behavior that alternates between extremes can throw you off kilter and compromise your sense of proportion and propriety.

You've probably had the same types of experiences. Family members and loved ones often find themselves trying to rescue people with BPD. After a particularly wonderful period with Sadie, Brad suddenly found himself writing a check for her poorly defined new business even though he was going to have to withdraw funds from his retirement account to cover it. Months into their marriage, Brad found out that Sadie's older sister had bailed her out of financial disasters for years, despite repeated vows never to help her again. Sadie's mother was under strict doctor's orders to find a way to reduce the stress that was draining her but could not bring herself to let the phone ring when she knew it was Sadie calling in the middle of the night, even when it was the third or fourth time in an hour, as it often was. People who love someone with BPD often give money, time, support, and so much of their concern that they become fatigued. Sometimes they reach the point where the relationship feels intolerable. Many, many people with BPD have lost most or all of the people in their lives. Or their social and family circle seems to be fitted with one big revolving door by which people exit and then return, over and over.

Maybe you're familiar with this scenario: You're in a room with your loved one who has BPD. You're having a great time, and it seems pretty clear that your loved one is too. There's a lot of laughter and sharing and mutual understanding. Your loved one—let's say it's your brother—goes home, and you're left with the glow of good will. Then all of a sudden, hours later, you get a phone call. It's your brother, and he's spewing out a list of all the things that you said and did that hurt him terribly. You're completely thrown. Were you two even in the same room together? Did you imagine the whole encounter? Were you that blind to the fact that your brother was upset at the time? No wonder you feel lost. You may also feel angry, defensive, confused, and guilty. So you react from your own emotions. Maybe you yell and hang up. Maybe you just withdraw, telling your brother you need a little time and distance.

This only makes things worse. Now you're getting multiple telephone calls from your brother, some with cursing and threats, some with tears and bewilderment, and many, many hang-ups. You withdraw more.

The next thing you find out is that your brother is in the psychiatric hospital following an overdose. He was trying to kill himself because he was so upset by your nonresponsiveness. You feel so guilty that you swear to your brother that you will *never* abandon him again.

But, of course that turns out to be an impossible promise to keep, because a few weeks later you are "hurting" your brother again ... and he is calling again.

Like Brad, you begin to feel like everything you do is wrong. Now you're constantly worried that your brother may kill himself the next time you upset him. And you start to feel a lot of resentment. You stay in the relationship, feeling like a yo-yo, bouncing back and forth between despair that your relationship is out of control and hope that things can be better. Many people who love someone with BPD feel like they're constantly losing their balance.

This sequence of events befalls almost everyone who is intimately involved with a person with BPD. It happens to therapists, family members, and friends. The relationships are terminated and begin again and are terminated again.

When you're closely involved with someone who has BPD, you may feel directionless, because all you can ever seem to do is react. You go from one extreme to the other, from trying to make sure nothing upsets the person you love to trying to get away from the person at all costs. You may feel like you're caught in a riptide, unsure when the behaviors that upset you are going to stop and where you're going to be dropped off at the end.

> *When your loved one's behavior requires attention, you can lose your sense of self-determination since all your time is spent reacting.*

At the same time, the relationship may be so intense that you can't find yourself in it at all. I probably don't have to tell you that relationships with those who have BPD are not typically characterized by quiet, easy companionship. Instead there's likely lots of high-intensity behavior that demands attention, accusations that cry out for an immediate defense, pleas that bring out the Lone Ranger in the least heroic of us.

I probably also don't have to tell you that the person with BPD has emotions that are like tornadoes. They can appear out of nowhere, gather strength, and wreak destruction. The emotional states of people with BPD change rapidly, and it's hard for the rest of us to keep up with them. It's emotion that's at the heart of the chaos. Because people with BPD often have no control over their emotions, they also seem to have very little control over their behavior. As you'll learn in this book, much of what they do—the impulsive decisions, the anger outbursts, the about-faces—is aimed at trying to deal with out-of-control, overwhelming emotion. The fact that you are either directly on the receiving end or on the cleanup crew has led many authors to say you have to protect yourself in relationships with emotionally sensitive people. They are accused of being full of rage (which sometimes they are), unpredictable (which they usually are), and volatile (which they definitely are). So, yes, it may very well make sense to protect yourself. But while you're doing so, it's also important to know that the extreme emotions and their accompanying behaviors are not usually a deliberate attempt to lose relationships, cause problems, or ruin anyone's life.

Understanding where these extreme emotions and their accompanying behaviors come from is a better antidote than simply protecting yourself. Lacking the knowledge that can reveal a better alternative often means that ending the relationship seems like the only solution. This book, therefore, is going to educate you about the nature of the behaviors that make up the diagnosis of BPD. Getting educated is the only way to have a relationship in which everyone can achieve better balance.

> When you're tired of unpleasant surprises, it's easy to lose your compassion.

*W*hat Does *Borderline Personality Disorder* Mean?

This is a difficult question to answer. Most people have an inkling of what *depression* means, or even something like *schizophrenia*. But what does *borderline* signify, and what's a *personality disorder*? Let's dispense with *borderline* just to get it out of the way. *Borderline* was a term created in the early 20th century, meant to indicate that this disorder fell in between two major classes of psychiatric diagnoses, neuroses and psychoses. That's all I'm going to say about it, because it's really irrelevant to your understanding of your loved one, though it does give you a hint at how tricky this disorder is to get a handle on and to diagnose. As to *personality disorder*, what you need to know about this term is that it means your loved one exhibits a chronic pattern of behaviors that are based in his or her personality, which means essentially that they affect everything: moods, actions, and relationships. You can probably see this pretty plainly for yourself.

To get into a little more detail, if you were to consult the *Diagnostic and Statistical Manual of Mental Disorders* (DSM-IV-TR; the manual that psychiatrists and other mental health professionals use as a guide for diagnosing BPD and other disorders), you would see nine diagnostic criteria listed. They range from suicidal and self-harm behaviors to psychotic behaviors to behaviors intended to avoid abandonment. These criteria are often cumbersome and difficult to pinpoint. Many mental health professionals have found it challenging to diagnose the disorder using these criteria, because they are so wide-ranging and because the disorder can manifest itself in such diverse ways. Maybe your loved one is dramatic, impulsive, and emotional, the profile that's pretty common and that I've been alluding to so far in this chapter. But your loved one could also qualify for the disorder if she often seems emotionless or numb (more on this a little later in the chapter). Some people with BPD function brilliantly as parents and friends but can't keep a job; others abuse alcohol and/or drugs and can't function normally in any domain of life. Unfortunately, I don't think the DSM criteria make it easy to see that these people all suffer from the same underlying problem.

I also think that the wording in the DSM makes BPD sound untreatable and fuels despondence in people with the diagnosis. The psychiatrist who diagnosed Sadie and only made Brad feel worse is a good case in point.

Dr. Marsha M. Linehan, originator of dialectical behavior therapy (DBT), the type of treatment I use to help people with BPD, thought that there had to be a better way to capture and identify what was going on in this disorder. So she reclassified the diagnosis into five areas of dysregulation. That is, she identified five different ways that people with BPD are unable to regulate themselves—their behavior, their emotions, their thoughts—the way other people do. Dividing the diagnostic "symptoms" into these subgroups of behaviors makes the behaviors of your loved one, and a lot of others with the disorder who may look vastly different on the surface, understandable and, even more important, treatable.

Being familiar with these subgroups can also make it a lot easier to understand why you feel so lost in your relationship. It may help you understand why you're having such a hard time deciding what you can do to improve your relationship while still being interested in preserving it. As you read about the five areas described below, ask yourself whether you see these problems in the person you love. I'm not asking you to undertake an amateur diagnosis, and I'm definitely not asking you to judge. Just look at the behaviors. The key is to try to keep some distance and observe the behaviors as if you were watching television. As difficult as it may be not to get embroiled in rehashing painful events, try not to jump into interpreting or blaming your loved one for the behaviors that seem to fit into these subgroups. Instead, just try to start noticing patterns. This is a first step toward regaining your balance and becoming "unlost."

Extra-Sensitive and Highly Reactive Emotions

Jill wakes up every morning and says to herself, "I am not going to over-react today." She goes downstairs to fix breakfast for her children and soon realizes they are not getting ready for school quickly enough, so she finds herself becoming irritated. At the school, she stops in to talk with one of the kids' teachers. The teacher says that her daughter is struggling in reading class. Jill feels very sad about her daughter and then begins to believe it is all her fault. Her shame and guilt build to the point that she needs to do something to feel better. She stops at the local department store and buys clothes that are on sale. When she gets home and realizes how much money she has spent, she is mortified. She begins to call herself names: "idiot, worthless." Jill turns on the TV and finds herself sobbing during a talk show. Finally, she pulls out a bottle of vodka. Just one glass will help make her feel better ...

As Jill exemplifies, people who suffer from *emotional dysregulation* are really at the mercy of their highly tuned emotional system all the time. I know, you undoubtedly feel like you're at its mercy too. Believe me, it's not pleasant for either of you. Emotional dysregulation can feel like drinking a cup of boiling coffee that everyone else insists is just lukewarm. Where you might feel a twinge of irritation, an emotionally dysregulated person feels instant rage. Where you feel a flush of attraction to someone, the person with BPD may feel irresistible desire. Something that makes you feel slightly embarrassed might send the emotionally dysregulated person scurrying off to cut herself repeatedly or drink a fifth of bourbon to obliterate the feeling of overwhelming shame.

It may not surprise you to know that emotional dysregulation is the primary area of dysregulation for people with BPD. In fact, the other four types of dysregulation either result from the fast, extreme emotions of the person with BPD or are an attempt to get relief or avoid the emotions.

When I say that people with BPD have "fast" emotions, I mean they come up quickly and change quickly. So suddenly, in fact, that you probably don't usually have any idea what has triggered an emotional change in your loved one because the trigger can be so subtle. In a short time, your wife or brother-in-law has flipped from laughing and seemingly happy to full of shame and then to anger and then to sadness. When I say that people with BPD have "extreme" emotions, I mean that they are typically very, very intense. What this adds up to for you is that your loved one's emotions seem unpredictable.

On his way out of a dinner party his sister-in-law gave, Mike smiles sincerely and thanks her for having him. Sandy immediately gets very upset and insulted. Mike is thrown: isn't it just good manners to thank someone for dinner? Awkwardly he tries to regroup, protesting that he doesn't understand Sandy's reaction. Sandy then gets even angrier, accusing Mike of "not understanding me." Mike gets more and more flustered, his mind racing as he tries to figure out what to say to keep Sandy from having a total meltdown in front of her friends and family. As he leaves, he feels terrible, blaming himself for saying the "wrong" thing and then answering himself mentally by blaming Sandy, whose intense reaction we call "emotional lability."

As you probably know from experience, it's the unpredictability that you can count on with emotional lability—when someone has extreme emotional reactions that are quick to change, you never know what exact reaction you're going to get. At another time, Mike's confusion at Sandy's initial anger might have evoked not more anger but instant self-loathing and shame as she realized that she'd done the wrong thing (again).

Shame, in fact, is enemy number one of people with BPD. It only reinforces from the inside the invalidation of their emotional experience that they are already getting from the outside. If your loved one has passed his or her twenties, you may see one particularly confusing product of shame and the catastrophic consequences of emotionality: times when your loved one seems to be emotionless. This is the result of learning. When young, the consequences of your loved one's intense, extreme emotions may repeatedly have been catastrophic: people who are emotionally sensitive lose relationships, get kicked out of social circles, and get fired from paid and volunteer work (once I knew a person whose Alcoholics Anonymous group moved its meeting location to get away from her). After a period of time, the person with BPD learns something like this: "Emotions are bad, and I shouldn't have them." So your loved one may have begun to overcontrol his emotions (vs. undercontrolling them when younger). He may actually look like he isn't having emotions when the event would warrant emotions. Of course, the problem is that he is shutting down or suppressing emotion, and ultimately those emotions will erupt, the result usually a big, problematic emotional event.

All of this emotional upheaval is very uncomfortable for many people who feel emotions less intensely. You may feel like you're losing control of your life if you're always on guard for the next outburst.

You may find it very difficult not to judge your loved one for lacking the kind of self-control everyone else seems to have. But if you simply identify emotional sensitivity as a characteristic instead of a character flaw, you might not feel so much like you're always at the mercy of your loved one's emotions—and you might feel less caught up by resentment that he or she isn't controlling those emotions when everyone else is expected to do so.

Problems Getting Along with Others

Shauna can't stop thinking about the fact that her sister canceled tomorrow's lunch date because her kindergartner is sick. She can't sleep because she's ruminating over whether her sister just made up an excuse so she wouldn't have to see her. Before long she's in tears, and she calls her sister without stopping to think about whether 4:00 A.M. is a good time to phone. Sobbing, she screams when her sister answers, "You're just never a good sister to me like I am to you! I hate you!" Her sister is used to this and gently says that Shauna *is* a good sister and that she, too, tries to be and will try harder in the future. She hangs up, but before her head hits the pillow Shauna has called back. This time her sister gets testy and tells her she can't talk until she gets some sleep. The third time Shauna calls, her sister picks up the phone and scolds Shauna before hanging up. Shauna tries one more time, but her sister doesn't answer because she's turned the phone off.

It's not hard to see why the DSM calls the group of problems demonstrated in these snapshots *interpersonal chaos*. People with BPD really struggle in relationships. They desperately want to have relationships. In fact they consider relationships the most important thing in the world, and they're intensely afraid that people will leave them. The reality is that people *have* left them; their fears are not unfounded.

So from the outside it's probably hard to believe that they keep doing the things that drive people away. Usually, however, that's because people with BPD really don't know how to act in relationships. And when you add a lack of interpersonal skills to emotional dysregulation, you definitely have a recipe for chaotic interactions with others.

Shauna's emotions were in overdrive when she phoned her sister. She felt so terrified of being abandoned by her sibling that she impulsively picked up the phone at a time when most people would know there's no way they'd get a positive, constructive reaction. She also doesn't have the interpersonal communication skills to tell her sister that her tone of voice when she canceled their plans made Shauna suspect she wasn't telling the truth, which hurt her. So instead, she blasted her sister for not being what she wants and needs. Her sister tried to get off the phone as quickly as possible (by placating, reacting angrily, and hanging up); she knew from experience that no good was going to come from trying to chat. Then Shauna got scared to death that she was going to lose her sister. She worried and panicked and kept calling, not realizing that this very behavior jeopardized her relationship with her sister and could actually bring about what Shauna feared most: that her sister would cut her out of her life.

Many people with BPD have great difficulty holding on to a job, rarely because they don't have the intelligence to perform all kinds of tasks. While Brad was doubting himself, his family and friends were trying to convince him that Sadie was "using" him. Close relatives of people who lose job after job often conclude that they are irresponsible, lazy, and manipulative, preferring to be supported financially by others rather than fulfill normal adult responsibilities. What they actually lack is the interpersonal skills that make civil and productive workplace relationships possible. If you know that your loved one may lack such skills and that the consequences of this deficit are huge when combined with emotional dysregulation, you may be able to suspend judgments that only widen the rift in your relationship.

Acting on Impulse—Even When It's Dangerous

Linda had had a rough day. She woke up on the wrong side of the bed. She had a migraine. She went to the emergency room to get help for the migraine, and the wait was four hours. The nurse was rude to her, and Linda felt like the hospital staff had treated her like a drug addict. She left the hospital before getting any help and went to the nearby casino instead. Linda lost all of the money that she had with her and some money she withdrew from the ATM at the poker table. She rented a hotel room, ordered a bottle of bourbon, and swallowed all the pills she had in her purse. She started talking very loudly to herself, so the hotel manager came to check on her. Linda ended up being taken to the emergency room again. This time in handcuffs.

Joe got into an argument with his manager. He went to his desk but was so angry that he couldn't concentrate. Instead he walked off his job.

Once Joe got into his car, he realized what he had done. Overcome with shame, he went to the closest bridge to jump.

Caroline is in college. She is beautiful, smart, and talented. However, she gets very anxious before tests. She will study for the test, but even if she knows the material her anxiety builds and builds. Right before the test, she cuts herself four or five times with a single-edge razor blade. Her anxiety becomes manageable.

If these stories sound familiar, you know that the third area of dysregulation is the one that instills the most fear in people who love someone with BPD. It's called *behavioral dysregulation*, and it's what causes people to act impulsively and repeatedly without seeming to learn from the negative consequences. Sometimes it seems like they never look before they take the proverbial leap into dangerous activities. Other times it is like they look but take the leap anyway. The impulsive behaviors may lead to your loved one sometimes ending up hospitalized, incarcerated, homeless, or penniless.

Acting on Impulse

If your loved one quits jobs or relationships, binges, purges, drinks, takes drugs, shoplifts, commits crimes, runs away, or does anything that is impulsive, he is engaging in dysregulated behavior. What drives these behaviors is that they very often serve to make the person feel better or at least to eliminate intense emotion. By engaging in these behaviors, your loved one can avoid or shut down emotions and provide himself with relief. The relief is, however, just temporary. The person feels better for a short time, but then new, painful emotions come up in response to the impulsive behaviors. These emotions are usually shame and guilt. They distress the person so much that she often has to shut them down, and a cycle begins. The urge to shut down painful emotion makes mind- and body-altering substances a typical resort of those with BPD. But so are self-destructive behaviors like cutting and other forms of self-harm, discussed below.

People with borderline personality seem to lose their judgment, especially when their emotions are high. In some ways it's easier to understand poor decision making under emotional duress than impulsive decision making. People with BPD may pursue an unwise love interest (like going home from a bar with a total stranger), spend lots of money, take off on a spontaneous trip, berate a boss or other authority figure, make those late-night phone calls, run away from home—whatever pops into their head (and sometimes it doesn't even really seem to be an idea before it is an action) and eases the uncomfortable emotion they happen to be feeling. As the impulsive behaviors work to relieve emotions over time, they become almost automatic responses to emotion. That is, people with BPD engage in the impulsive behavior before they fully experience the painful emotion and without making conscious decisions to engage in impulsive behavior.

Impulsive behavior is what we call *negatively reinforcing*: the behavior results in the shutting off of negative emotion. It is not that people with BPD don't learn from their mistakes, as is often said to be the case. The problem is that either the behavior that shuts the emotion down happens faster than decision making or the urge to relieve the discomfort of the emotion is stronger than anything else. If you remember, too, that these behaviors do serve a purpose, even if only briefly, it's easier to understand that people with BPD are not just obstinately refusing to catch on.

Unfortunately, when you're observing—and being affected by—impulsive behaviors that cause your loved one such trouble, you can end up feeling helpless and lost in chaos. You want to understand and help, and yet your spouse or sibling just keeps shooting him- or herself in the foot. DBT gives people with BPD the skills they need to start acting in their own best interests. Meanwhile, there are things you can do to make yourself feel more grounded, as detailed in later chapters.

Suicide Attempts and Other Self-Harm

It's a harsh and horrifying fact that many people with BPD make multiple suicide attempts. They also engage in self-harming behaviors that are not an attempt to kill themselves (cutting themselves, scratching themselves, burning themselves, pulling out stitches). These behaviors are really frightening. For those who love them, it's essential to know that just because BPD causes some people to engage in nonsuicidal self-harm, this does *not* mean they won't also try to commit suicide. Contrary to the popular lore of recent years that people with BPD don't kill themselves—they are just "manipulating" or "acting out" and will not die—around 10% of people with BPD do die by suicide (suicide is a major risk for these people, and 11% of those who begin by cutting end up dead by suicide). Because it's a reality you have to deal with, I'll

Suicide does occur in those with BPD. Cutting and other self-harm behaviors are not always suicide attempts.

devote Chapter 12 to this difficult topic. For now, though, it may help to understand why it's such a common impulse among people with BPD.

Self-harm is a case where another area of dysregulation is meant to provide relief from the primary area, emotional dysregulation. Sometimes something happens to a person with BPD that triggers excruciating emotions. The emotions build and build until the person literally thinks she might burst with the pain. The person with BPD may end up believing that suicide is the only way to stop that emotional pain. Sometimes just thinking or fantasizing about killing herself (or just being dead) makes the intense emotion go down. There is actually research data suggesting that suicidal behaviors, including thinking about being dead, provide real, physical relief from intense emotional states. The same is true with other self-harm behaviors. They work to calm intense emotional states. This, of course, applies to all of us. The difference is that people with BPD have a much greater need for the relief that self-harm can provide because of their heightened emotional sensitivity; also, many times they don't have the skills to use more effective behaviors to get relief.

Sometimes people resort to suicidal or self-harm behaviors to prevent painful emotions from arising at all. If your loved one has learned to take this course of action, the suicidal/self-harm response may become almost automatic: something happens, and immediately the person engages in suicidal or self-harm behaviors, seemingly without thinking about it. This reflex to harm oneself may seem downright bizarre. Most of us can understand, at least in theory, the urge to shut down intolerable pain. But the idea that someone would go directly to self-harm following a certain event, without even experiencing the pain of the event, may seem unfathomable. This is why it's so important to understand your loved one's internal experience—you can feel adrift in some kind of surreal universe if you observe these behaviors and try to interpret them in the context of your own very different but more typical internal experience.

When you're trying to understand suicidal behaviors in your loved one, it's particularly important to avoid the judgmental idea that these actions are intended to manipulate you or someone else. Sometimes people with BPD (and others) do engage in suicidal behaviors to get a response from others. But they're not always aware of it. And even when they are, they have not usually plotted to do this to get your sympathy. Remember that more often than not the person is acting on an impulse. Also keep in mind that if your loved one doesn't have interpersonal skills to call on in getting help, she can see a lot fewer options for easing her own pain.

A few weeks ago, a client of mine was at home alone and bored. She was very lonely and feeling ignored by her mother, who was taking care of a sick child with special needs. My client cut herself deeply several times on her legs and ended up in the local emergency room. When the client and I talked about her behavior, she said that she had cut herself with the intention of relieving boredom. She also wanted to "show Mom that she needed to pay some attention to me too."

I had another client who believed her husband was very critical of her. As we began to look at patterns in her suicidal behavior, she and I discovered that following her overdoses her husband would quit criticizing her for a period of time. Harming herself to stop the criticism was not a part of her overt decision making, but her behavior *was* changing the behavior of her husband. This can be a tough distinction to grasp. It's hard for most of us to understand that someone can behave in a way that is followed by a certain response without having intentionally tried to elicit that response. However, all animals do this. If a child stays home from school because he's sick and you give him his favorite food treat, there is a chance that he will be sick more often. He isn't thinking, "Hmmm, if I stay home from school, Mom will give me ice cream." His sick days just multiply. If I take my husband to see action movies (which he loves) every time he finishes a household project, he will begin to finish household projects more often. It may not be in his awareness that he is finishing the projects to get to see the movies, but the projects do get finished over time.

What's important to understand is that self-harm behaviors are learned. Suicide is not a behavioral response that we are born with. Somewhere, somehow, your loved one learned that suicidal or self-harm behaviors work for her. It could be that the behavior regulates emotion (as for the client whose cutting relieved her boredom) or that it has a desired effect on the behaviors of others (as for the woman whose husband would take a hiatus from criticizing her). Or it might stop the person from "zoning out" (dissociating, defined below). Whatever the "benefit," you're probably thrown by the idea that anyone would consider self-harm a good way to solve any problem. You may have agonized many times over why your loved one would take such drastic actions, which are so obviously (to you) a bad way to solve any problem. It may help you regain your sense of balance if you keep in mind that self-harm is just a form of behavioral dysregulation, like impulsively quitting jobs or getting intimately involved with strangers. The good news is that learned behavior can be unlearned and replaced with healthier choices—one of the goals of DBT.

Loss of a Sense of Self, or Self-Dysregulation

I once worked with a person who could not tell me whether she preferred chocolate or vanilla ice cream. I took her to an ice cream shop for a scoop, and she could not make a decision. When I asked, "What do you like?" her sincere response was "I don't know." Most of us don't even have to think about such trivial preferences. People with BPD often don't have a sense of what they like, what their values are, or who they are.

I've had other clients whose intimate relationships were always short-lived or chaotic because they did not know what they wanted in relationships or because they thought there was no reason anyone would want to stay in a relationship with them. The clients don't know what kind of partner they want. Many times they are not sure what their sexual preferences are. They are empty and look to others to help fill the void, yet they struggle with believing they deserve anything other than emptiness. One of my clients once described himself as a bucket with holes in the bottom. Nothing would help him feel anything other than empty.

> How could people with no awareness of personal preferences begin to understand who they really are?

Most of us have at least some idea of who we are and what our place is in the world. We have roles; we have a sense of our values; we know what we like and don't like. We have dreams and goals. People with BPD do not have a sense of who they are. In the moment, they are unable to identify what their experience is—what they feel in their bodies, what their thoughts and emotions are. They often judge themselves very harshly and struggle to develop realistic goals for their future. They do not know their values or their likes and dislikes.

Not knowing who you are is a byproduct of the extreme emotionality of people with BPD. People who are having intense emotions most of the time cannot pay attention to their internal experiences and reactions to situations. It's like trying to read a road sign in the middle of a hurricane. The road sign is spinning and spinning. You know it is a road sign, but you don't know what it says. People with BPD know that there are values and preferences, but they can't read them because of the emotions that are interfering. Because they can't grasp who they are, they feel lost and empty. Feeling lost and empty increases their shame—and so on.

Because the woman who didn't know what ice cream flavor she preferred had no sense of self, she made impulsive decisions; she had no core beliefs or values or personal preferences to guide her. Because she had no sense of self, she, like so many others with BPD I have known, thought there was no reason for anyone to want to be in a relationship with her—she didn't know what her positive attributes were. Of course, this affected her relationship stability, which caused her to be more emotional, make more impulsive decisions, and worry about why people would stay in her life.

What Could They Be Thinking?

"What were you *thinking?*" is something you may have asked your loved one time and time again. Baffling behavior, emotional reactions, interpersonal gaffes, and a lot of doubt about who they are can leave onlookers flabbergasted by the way people with BPD lead their lives. The answer to your question is that your loved one may very well not be thinking exactly the same way you do. The final area of dysregulation is what we call *cognitive dysregulation*. As with the other areas, this type of dysregulation can take different forms in different people at different times.

Trouble Paying Attention

In one form, people with cognitive dysregulation have a very difficult time controlling their attention. Because emotions interfere with anyone's ability to concentrate, the big emotions of people with BPD cause them to have trouble concentrating. Think about a time when you were really emotional about something. Maybe you tried to talk with someone or even watch television. You couldn't follow the conversation or the television show. Your emotions were affecting your ability to concentrate.

Some (not all) people with BPD may automatically do what we call *dissociating*. There are a lot of scientific descriptions of dissociation, but you can think of dissociating informally as "zoning out." If you've ever driven home and then realized you were not paying attention at all and didn't really remember how you got home, you did some low-level dissociating. We all dissociate to some degree. People who dissociate often do so in the presence of something that triggers extreme emotional reactions, such as talking about something painful or being in a place that triggers memories of a painful event.

Sometimes people with BPD describe dissociation as "shutting down." At times it may be apparent that your loved one is dissociating because she becomes expressionless and still and her vocal tone may become flat. It will appear that she is not fully present. Other times, the dissociation may be so subtle that you don't notice it. Dissociation, like cutting and self-harm behaviors, provides relief from intense emotional experiences. It's like throwing up a wall between the painful stimulus and your loved one. The problem is that it is temporary and that your loved one is not experiencing emotions. We all have to experience emotions to live functional lives.

Paranoia

People with BPD can actually have moments when they are paranoid. Usually the paranoia is wrapped into extreme emotionality and interpersonal chaos. Your loved one may appear to be preoccupied with whether or not you are about to leave him. This, of course, makes him more emotional, makes him more fearful and convinced that you are going to leave, and causes him to seek confirmation that your behavior indicates you were planning to leave. You actually were not thinking about leaving, but naturally you react to being told that you did have this nefarious scheme. You become emotional under the weight of being accused unjustly, and your loved one uses this as "evidence" that you are leaving. The cycle continues. You actually do begin to question why you are with this person who does not trust you or the relationship. Second-guessing yourself in this way can naturally make you feel lost. So can the fact that at times of duress the person with BPD may get so suspicious or fearful that others are out to get him that he seems to have lost touch with reality. You may start to worry that your loved one has a psychotic disorder (such as schizophrenia). But when the trigger of the paranoia goes away (the family reunion is over, for example), so does the paranoia. Or when the general life stressors of the person with BPD decrease, the paranoia subsides along with them. This is usually an enormous relief, but you still may live in fear of the next episode. The important thing to remember is that the paranoia is short-lasting and stress induced. The high emotionality of your loved one in stressful situations may make him overly suspicious.

$\mathcal{D}$o You See How All These Patterns of Behaviors Relate?

Maybe you can now see how the five areas of dysregulation interact to create some pretty baffling behavior. Perhaps you can consider the possibility that your loved one isn't acting "crazy" on purpose, just to elicit some reaction from you, but is being carried along on this roller coaster herself. Feeling emotions intensely and not knowing how to regulate them can lead to desperate actions to ease pain. The fallout of those desperate acts can leave your loved one terrified of being rejected at work or abandoned in love. Having difficulty concentrating and learning fully from mistakes may cause a person with BPD to attack in anticipation of being hurt—leading to a self-fulfilling prophecy of abandonment. Abandonment causes more pain and also confirms the person's sense of worthlessness. Without a sense of self, the person continues to flail about, trying out new partners, new jobs, new friends to see if anything or anyone fits and can help define who she is. It's a cycle that's clearly destructive, and yet without an understanding of what drives it, it's a cycle that's hard to break. DBT can help your loved one understand what's going on and begin to regulate those emotions and subsequent behaviors. Adopting some of its principles and responding to your loved one in new ways based on your understanding of the five areas of dysregulation can help you regain your balance and find a way to preserve your relationship.

What Makes Someone So Emotional?

BPD is complicated. At its core, it's an emotional problem. But radiating out from a supersensitive emotional system are problems with all aspects of daily living. Because they have so much trouble regulating their emotions, people with BPD often have shaky relationships. They act without thinking, and even when they do think they often can't figure out the effective thing to do. They're distracted and sometimes paranoid. They don't really know themselves, what to do or say, what's fact and what's their interpretation of the facts. Naturally it's hard to predict their direction or destination or to know when they're going to veer off, crash into something, and fall apart. Agonizing, out-of-control emotions cause pervasive life problems, and the result is usually chaos.

Why, then, wouldn't your loved one just do what's necessary to get those emotions under control and banish chaos from her life (and yours)?

Because it's just not that simple. People with BPD are born with a particular vulnerability to emotion, the same way some people are born with red hair or dark skin or a talent in music, sports, or math. They can't just turn off their emotions any more than they can change their eye color or trade in a tin ear for perfect pitch. As they grow up, their innate emotional sensitivity not only causes them pain on the inside but also meets with a lot of intolerance (even disbelief) from those on the outside. Through interwoven pathways that I want to map in this chapter, they end up lacking a lot of the skills that the rest of us develop without much conscious effort while growing up.

Fortunately, they can still learn these skills, which is the precise focus of DBT. Insisting that people with BPD "get control over their emotions" doesn't work, as you've probably seen. In fact it often makes things worse, because being reminded that there's something "wrong" with them brings up painful emotions all by itself. DBT provides an alternative in the form of specific skills that help them maintain good relationships, tolerate distress and survive crises, and learn to use their emotions as the important resource they were designed to be. Emotional control actually follows, as you'll see if your loved one is receiving DBT.

> Being told to "get control over their emotions" only increases emotions, especially shame, in people with BPD, and shame is an emotion most find impossible to bear.

Even if she isn't getting this type of therapy, what you'll learn in this book will give *you* ways to help her stay out of the emotional vortex without demanding she do the impossible and shrug off the inborn traits of emotional vulnerability. Meanwhile, I think you'll find that using these skills eases your own stress and frustration by helping to keep your emotions on an even keel too.

*H*ardwired to Be Highly Emotional

It takes two basic ingredients and time to make BPD. The first ingredient is an innate, biological vulnerability to emotions. Think of it as being hardwired for how we experience emotions. Each of us is born to feel emotion with a certain degree of intensity. You might not be used to viewing emotions this way. Some people believe we all experience emotions the same way, to the same degree. They believe even people who seem to feel emotions more intensely than others are simply exerting less self-control than those around them. But we know from scientific study that how much emotion each person feels, how often, is not a matter of choice. Observations of how newborn babies respond to different tests in hospital nurseries tell us that individual human beings have varying emotional responses well before learning has a chance to shape them. In one such test, infants were tickled on their noses with feathers. Some babies had almost no emotional response (they did nothing), some babies had a mild emotional response (they moved around), and some babies began crying and were hard to console. The babies who had an intense emotional response were then viewed as being "sensitive to emotional stimuli"—they reacted more quickly and more intensely to experiences that tend to evoke some kind of emotion. So, from birth, we apparently have an encryption for how we experience emotions.

If you think about children you know, you'll see there's lots of support for this theory. We start describing kids' emotional temperament early in their lives, calling some babies "fussy" and others "easy." Parents often marvel at the unique dispositions that their offspring display right from day one—little Johnny being so different from older sister Jenny. What we are really talking about is the child's early emotional responses.

Think about your own family or even a group of close friends. You probably expect certain types of emotional reactions from each person. Whether it's talking about something as mundane as where to go out for dinner or something as critical as what to do about Great-aunt Emma's worsening Alzheimer's disease, Cindy always knows how a family confab will go: Her husband, Bud, will sit there placidly, showing no emotional reaction to anything but giving well-thought-out assessments when asked to weigh in. Her irrepressible sister Georgia will laugh and make light of even the most serious statements. Mom will have to leave the room when anyone starts to bicker. Dad will get loudly angry if he feels like anyone has shown him disrespect. Some people have many emotions, all of them strong. Some people have very few emotions. Some people seem to have a balance of emotions. There are people who feel certain emotions very intensely and others mildly.

People with BPD have an exquisite vulnerability to emotions, meaning they are the babies in the nursery who have an extreme response to getting tickled on the nose with feathers. If you grew up with the person in your life who has BPD, I am sure your memory is of a child you'd describe as "emotional." Unfortunately, that general term doesn't tell you much that can help you understand and live with the person today. But if we tease apart this emotionality, it becomes easier to see that being "emotional" is not really a lack of control as much as three separate tendencies that cause emotional arousal in different ways.

Emotional Sensitivity: A Quick Trigger Finger

I was with someone the other night who came into my office calmly, without any apparent emotional discomfort. She said she really had only one question to discuss. She was trying to figure out whether she should quit her job as a high school art teacher in the middle of the school year. As we began to discuss it, I tried to help her figure out what we needed to look at to solve the problem. Did she want to quit teaching? Did she not want to teach art? What were the repercussions of quitting during a contracted school year? She became very angry at me. I stopped. I told her that I was there to do what she needed and tried to return to figuring out exactly what the problem was and to tell her I understood how she felt and which parts of her experience made sense and were wise. She became even angrier. When I asked her if she was angry because I did not understand her problem, she said that she was not. She was angry because I *did* understand her problem and that meant she was stupid, because it took me a short amount of time to figure it out. I tried to tell her that it's easier on the outside sometimes and that it's frustrating to try to figure out what to do with problems. Then she became despondent and teary. It seemed that no matter what I did, my responses were wrong and functioned to make her angrier and more upset. Finally, I said, "I just don't know what to say here. I'm trying to be helpful and give you some hope, but it's not working. What do you want me to do to help you?" At which point she exploded and said that she had come in to get me to answer one question and I was not doing my job.

This is what emotional sensitivity can look like from the outside. Things that trigger little or no emotion in most people trigger huge emotions in those with BPD. People with BPD are often described as "wearing their heart on their sleeve" or "being just too sensitive." They react emotionally to any trigger, whether it is with what we consider the "negative" emotions (fear, sadness, anger, shame, guilt) or the more "positive" emotions (joy, happiness, love). Whether your loved one is having positive or negative emotions, the fact that you wouldn't have an emotional reaction to whatever just set off your loved one's emotions can make it really hard for you to identify the trigger at all, so you may often feel blindsided. In that case you'll probably be interested to know that your loved one may be just as confused by this sensitivity as you are. The person with BPD often is unsure why he is having such an emotional reaction and struggles to contain it. Meanwhile, you're having the surreal experience that there are two extremely different stories about what is happening or has happened.

I just told you the story that was unfolding in my office from my point of view. After my client's emotions had subsided and we were able to move on, I heard her story: She had walked into my office early to find me writing an e-mail. She came in saying she was 5 minutes early. I motioned for her to sit down and asked her to let me finish a sentence in the message I was sending. Although I still started the session with her a few minutes early, she had been terribly injured that I did not stop writing the e-mail and begin her session instead of finishing and sending it. But at the time that her emotions were overtaking her, my client said, she had had no idea what was setting them all off, and the more emotions she had, the more intense they were and the more emotions they raised.

It's important to understand that people having this kind of experience can't just turn off their emotions because they "make no sense." It's easy to believe that if they can't put their finger on the reason they're feeling the way they do, it must be because there is no reason—and that once this is pointed out to them they should easily be able to stop feeling the emotion. It doesn't work that way. The fact that the trigger is unnameable doesn't mean it doesn't exist.

> To understand emotional sensitivity, think of the person with BPD as being "raw." His emotional nerve endings are exposed, and so he is acutely affected by anything emotional.

Have you ever had a time when your loved one was really upset about something (or at you) and you had absolutely no idea what the upset was about? The husband of someone I know described the experience this way: "I thought my wife was upset about my coming home late, because that's the first thing she said, but she kept changing her mind, and finally she admitted she had no idea why she was so upset but just felt like she was going to jump out of her skin she was so angry; then she collapsed in tears."

If you've ever been with someone with BPD, thinking everything was going fine, only to get a phone call 2 hours later and hear that the person is very distressed and how upset she is by what you did, you have witnessed emotional sensitivity. Sometimes the person appears to be fine in the moment or really is fine. Then, later, she plays back the time with you and in doing so begins to react, either to the conversation, to her interpretation of her behavior or yours, or to her own subsequent reactions ("I underreacted"). Any of these can be part of sensitivity. Emotional sensitivity wires people to react to cues and to react to their reactions. Sometimes the person seems to become distressed for no reason that you can see. The problem is that this leaves you confused, and now you don't trust your experiences either—one of the ways you end up feeling lost that we discussed in Chapter 1. Over time you don't trust that there will not be a reaction to something you are about to say or something you did say. You begin to sensor the information you give your loved one. You can actually feel some fear when you have to discuss something that you predict will cause an emotional reaction from the person. This puts stress on the relationship and can, over time, bring about the relationship's end.

- *People with borderline personality disorder can't change how much emotion they feel.*
- *Your loved one is probably just as confused as you are about what sets off her emotions.*
- *Not having a "good reason" for an intense emotional reaction doesn't make it easy to stop the emotion.*

Emotional Reactivity: Over the Top in Intensity

I once had a client who was very easily aroused to heights of emotion. She had been in many different types of therapy where the therapist had tried to help her understand why she had such a quick emotional trigger. Therapists couldn't get to the heart of her reactions because she reacted to everything as if it were criticism. In therapy with me, as in other therapies, she would get upset with me and storm out. Of course, she had the same over-the-top emotional reactions in her personal life. She would get distressed and storm out of her house, leaving her husband and children behind. Then she would drive around for hours, thinking about whether she should kill herself. On three occasions she checked into hotels, took an overdose of medication, and drank a lot of gin. Finally her relationship with her husband was destroyed. She then moved into her parents' house, and the same thing happened with them. Ultimately the client's leaving the house and the worries that her parents had about whether or not she was going to kill herself destroyed her relationship with her mother, who shortly afterward died suddenly.

Now this client suffers because she does not have a relationship with her family and because she was estranged from her mother when she died. Her shame and grief cause her to have even more big emotional reactions.

People like this woman are not only emotionally very sensitive to cues; they also have reactions that are very strong, more intense than for the average person. What would be sadness in most becomes overwhelming despair. What would be anger becomes rage. What would be embarrassment becomes humiliation. The intensity of the emotion is out of proportion, and, usually, so is the expression of it (your loved one may go to bed for days, cry in public, scream, and yell). This is what we call *emotional reactivity*.

You've probably caught yourself wondering sometimes why your loved one makes such a big deal out of what you view as unremarkable situations. What you are questioning is your loved one's reactivity. As with emotional sensitivity, you can end up affected by the extreme emotional responses. How do you respond to them? Do you withdraw from your loved one? Do you avoid talking about or doing things that might upset her? Do you worry about what her responses will be? If so, you're caught up in worries about the reactivity of your loved one, and as discussed in Chapter 1, the consequence is that you can end up feeling very lost in the relationship.

I'll give you some alternative responses that will ease your own discomfort and help preserve the relationship starting in Chapter 3. For now, though, it's helpful to try to remind yourself that, as with sensitivity, emotional reactivity is not self-indulgence or an attempt to "manipulate." New research evidence is beginning to suggest that what we have always thought of as heightened sensitivity in those with BPD is actually a higher emotional baseline. This would mean that if most people's basic emotional state is 20 on a 0- to 100-point scale, the person with BPD is always at an 80. It would mean your loved one may be in a constant state of emotional arousal and therefore is primed to have emotional responses to anything, great or small. A situation that would cause others to go from 20 to 30 on a 0- to 100-point scale makes your loved one go from 80 to 90. She is almost at the most extreme ends of emotionality.

To some extent emotional reactivity is a result of expecting the worst. People with borderline personality disorder are used to being rejected. They're used to making lots of mistakes. So any tiny reminder of a time when everything went wrong may bring on the same emotion—particularly deep shame or furious anger or one followed by the other—even though the situation at hand doesn't seem to warrant such an extreme response.

> Think for a moment how difficult it must be to **always** feel emotionally on edge.

Let's look a little more closely at anger in people with BPD. A typical view of those with the disorder is that they have "rage attacks," the implication being that their anger is totally unjustified—that it's wrong for them to feel the way they do. When you can't see what has set off the anger, it's understandable that you might believe there's something "wrong" with the whole emotional experience. And there's no doubt that people with BPD do have problems with anger. However, I don't see the problem as being whether or not they experience anger. I see the problem as lying in how intensely they experience the anger and how catastrophic the consequences of the anger often are to those with BPD and the people who love them.

After all, we all experience anger. Think of the last time you were stuck in traffic for an extended period of time. Was your blood boiling? How about the last time you felt you were treated unjustly? Anger can be a functional emotion. It helps motivate us to make needed changes in our lives, for one thing. Anger's positive function can be easy to forget, however, when your loved one seems to get so angry so often that you begin to believe she shouldn't have this emotion at all. This would be unfair to expect of anyone, of course.

So it's not your loved one's experiencing anger that is the problem. The problem is the intensity of the emotional reactions. If a supervisor at work came up to me and said something insensitive about my cat having died, I would definitely feel some emotion, probably some anger. But a person with BPD might become so angry that he would curse at the supervisor, call him a jerk, and then cry uncontrollably.

These extreme emotional reactions make it very difficult for people with BPD to be in relationships with others. Most of us simply don't do well when faced with extreme emotional reactions. We've learned to expect a certain level of emotional response to certain events. We can accept individual differences to a degree, but when someone's reactions exceed our expectations, it feels like an imposition: Is this person expecting us to do something to solve the problem that's causing all this emotion? Why does this person depart from the social conventions that

say you don't scream at your boss for being a little tactless or start sobbing because a stranger can't find his car in the parking lot? The rest of
us wouldn't dare act like that. There's no getting around the reality that
calling one's boss a jerk can have pretty self-destructive consequences,
and the person with BPD has to deal with that fallout. You, however,
can remind yourself that your loved one isn't being intentionally out of
control and inconsiderate when her emotional reactions are way out of
proportion; he just doesn't have the skills to keep his naturally high-
powered emotional engine from running away with him.

For a moment, put yourself in your loved one's shoes: You have huge
emotions that fire all the time. Your anger can be out of control. You
have lost jobs, lost friends, lost family, and lost your life goals because of
your emotions and mostly because of anger. What is a natural response
to all of this? You are frustrated, mostly with yourself. You judge yourself
as "stupid" or "defective." The consequence of all of your loss and judgments: you are even more emotional.

This is what happens with people with BPD. Most of them know
their emotions are out of control, and this insight causes even more
emotion—often shame or guilt. On top of the original anger, these
secondary emotions feel intoler-
able, and their fear of all this
emotion, ironically, tends to fire
off another series of emotions—
perhaps anger that is now shifted
to you, for "not helping" your
loved one or for some unex-
pressed reason. Lacking the ability to control these emotions,
your loved one may collapse in
tears, rush off somewhere as if it
were possible to leave the emo-

> - The fact that your loved
>   one's emotions are harmfully
>   intense doesn't mean that the
>   emotion is "wrong."
> - People with BPD aren't
>   purposely out of control
>   when they overreact; they
>   have no idea how to tone
>   down emotions that for them
>   are naturally intense.

tions behind physically, or make a desperate attempt to shut them down
through self-harm (as described in Chapter 1). You're left standing there,
wondering what hit you.

Slow Return to Baseline: Emotions That Overstay
Their Welcome

The third area of emotional vulnerability for people with BPD is a phys-
iologically slow return to baseline emotion. Not only do they react to

typically no-sweat events and react with an intensity that bowls others over, but they can't calm back down for a long time. Physically, the emotion fires for longer in the brain than with others. In a person with average emotional intensity, an emotion fires in the brain for around 12 seconds. There is evidence that in people with BPD emotions fire for 20% longer. So think about an emotion that you had that was intense. Think how long it took for you to quit having that emotion. Then think about having it for 20% longer than you had it. Now think about another emotion firing before that original emotion subsided and the second emotion staying around longer. And so on.

The person with BPD stays upset for an extended period of time. And, of course, the person acts upset and says upsetting things to others—blaming himself or others or expressing extreme despair and self-loathing. If you're on the receiving end, it's pretty natural to act on being upset. And as I bet you know, there's almost no reaction you can have that doesn't seem to drive your loved one's emotions back up to the top of the thermometer, including having no reaction.

Lisa was waiting for a date to pick her up, but he never came. She was very hurt. She was curled up in a ball on the sofa crying when her mother came in. Her mother tried to commiserate and tell her that she understood how painful it is to be stood up by a man. Lisa cried harder and told her mother that she couldn't possibly understand. She was just starting to calm down when her father walked in. The tears returned. When Dad began to say that the guy was a jerk and didn't deserve her, Lisa became angry and began defending the man. The event just didn't seem to end. Nothing Lisa's parents did could get her to calm down.

From the outside, unfortunately, you can't see that your loved one is trapped on an out-of-control roller coaster that she never intended to get on. What it may look like to you is that you're constantly inept at helping your loved one. Sometimes people make the judgment that those with BPD really enjoy being out of control and therefore keep that roller coaster careening along no matter what you say or do. I'll tell you more about how to get off that roller coaster yourself in Chapter 4, but one thing that sometimes works is just to give your loved one the time to get those emotions down by holding off on reacting at all for a moment. The woman in my office who heard everything as criticism and got more and more upset no matter what I said finally began to feel her emotions subside when I just got quiet.

A client came into my office a few weeks ago and told me that he had been so mad at me since the previous session that he had spent the entire week alternating between planning to drop out of therapy and planning to kill himself "just to show you how mad I really am!" What struck me about his anger is that he experienced it for an entire week. I know that for anger to last that long he had to have refired the emotion. As I said earlier, emotions last about 12 seconds, but they can stick around if they're reignited in the brain. Think about someone who cuts you off in traffic. You can be angry at him 2 hours later if you keep prompting the anger by thinking "That jerk. I can't believe he did that." Or, every time you see a car, the anger can fire off again without your doing anything to make it happen.

The way we do that with anger is to have thoughts about the person who has made us angry. We've all done this—rehashed some insult and gotten mad all over again. I am sure this man spent a great deal of time during the week perseverating about what I had said. But his emotions were high all week because of the event that occurred during our session. This is what happens: Emotions soar because of something that happens (you get cut off in traffic), and then you are sensitive to thoughts and cues ("What a jerk" or seeing sedans) that intensify your emotion, which then makes you sensitive to those cues ("He meant to do that" or few parking places at work), and so on. When I questioned the client, he could say that he did not, literally, experience nothing but anger at me during his week, but that when he did, he had the experience of being angry at me for hours and repeatedly. There were many things that set off his anger at me again that week. I had given him homework to do for our therapy session. Every time he looked at the paper with the homework assignment on it, his anger ignited. He heard someone say my first name, which is not an uncommon name, and his anger went up. At night when he went to bed, he would lie in bed and think about how angry he was at me. The cues for his anger were external (hearing someone with my name, seeing the homework sheets) and internal (thoughts of me, memories of the session), but they all worked to build the emotion over the week. The emotion became unbearable enough that he thought he could not

- If you think of "average" emotional experience as a wave with rolling ups and downs, the emotions of the person with BPD are all high peaks.
- Having emotions that keep going is like being on a runaway train. People with BPD don't want to keep that train going; they just don't know how to make it stop.

return to see me because he could not tolerate the overwhelming emotion of walking into a room with me.

Emotional Vulnerability Hurts

I want you to do something here that will help you understand what it's like to be extremely emotionally vulnerable. Think about a time when things were not going well in your life and you were having many emotions. For me, there was a time a few years ago when the company I worked for was going bankrupt, I was not sleeping, and everyone involved was really upset. I felt right on the edge of my emotions. Then a friend died. At that point I felt like every emotion that I had was at the surface of my skin. I physically felt like I would explode with emotion if one more thing happened. I did not want sympathy or understanding, because I was afraid that if anyone said something kind or understanding to me I would fall apart. It was very easy for me to become angry at anyone for anything. I was fearful about my future and sad about my friend. I was an emotional sponge. *One day in the midst of all of that emotion, when my skin literally hurt from all of the emotional pain, I realized that this was the experience of my clients with BPD every single day of their lives.*

So, think about the most emotional you have been for the longest period of time. Remember what it felt like emotionally and physically. Remember how it felt like emotions were just building on each other. Remember the experience of no one understanding how bad the situation was and how emotional you were. *Now tell yourself that this is the experience of your loved one every moment of every day.*

You may not want to recall such a painful period in your life every time you feel yourself losing your patience with your loved one. If so, try this image: Being in the thrall of emotional vulnerability is like not being able to find your keys and being frantic to get in your car and go. You have to be somewhere, you've looked everywhere for your keys, and you're getting more and more crazed. You have no idea what to do next and feel like you're about to explode. That's BPD from the inside.

The reality is that for people with BPD emotions are so intense, fire so easily, and last so long that they are miserable. Often people with BPD find ways to bring the emotion down. Cutting, suicide attempts, drinking, drugging, bingeing, purging, and other behaviors that can be problematic function to bring emotion down rapidly and to give relief. No wonder people with BPD engage in these behaviors. They work! To you, the damage done by these behaviors is so glaringly obvious that it may seem unbelievable that your loved one engages in them. But the fact that they ease pain at the moment makes it very difficult to get people to give them up.

Here's the thing. There are lots of us in the world who are emotionally sensitive. We are the ones who cry during television commercials, who laugh easily, who experience great joy (the upside of emotional sensitivity). We are usually very empathic because we can readily experience the emotions of others. But we do not all have BPD. So, being emotional is not the only thing that is required to make BPD. The other part is an invalidating environment.

*A*n Invalidating Environment

Emotional vulnerability is the first ingredient in the recipe for BPD. The second ingredient is an invalidating environment, and time is what pulls the two ingredients together. So when we talk about an invalidating environment that contributes to the emergence of BPD, we generally mean the environment in which the person grew up.

It's at this point in my explanation that those in the immediate family of people with BPD usually sigh, because they believe that this is where I tell them it is their fault that their relative—offspring, spouse, sibling—has BPD. I don't make that judgment, and neither should you. Parents and partners and brothers and sisters all do the best they can, and living with an emotionally sensitive person is not easy. An invalidating environment can be many things, as you'll see.

None of us is born knowing what to do with emotions. We are born with our capacity for emotional experiencing but not with the ability to do anything with emotions. We learn how to regulate emotions, a multifaceted process defined toward the end of this chapter, as we grow. The people in our environment show us through their own actions how to handle emotions. Some family members explicitly instruct kids about what to do with emotions, and some do not. Children who are less emotional need less direction in handling emotions, and children who are very emotional need a lot of help in learning how to deal with their emotionality.

For varying reasons, some family environments do not respond to the child as he or she needs. We call this an invalidating environment. The psychological definition of an invalidating environment is an environment where the responses of the child are pervasively treated as inaccurate, unrealistic, trivial, or pathological, independent of the actual validity of the behavior. This is really a mess of words, but here are some examples of invalidating responses:

The child says he doesn't like green beans. "Of course you like green beans. Everybody likes green beans."

The child brings home a grade of 98 on a test. "Why didn't you get a 100? I know you could have gotten a 100."

The child says she is hungry. "You are not hungry. You just ate."

The child comes home crying after a fight with a friend. "You didn't need him as a friend anyway."

The teenager comes home after a terrible day at high school. "Don't you complain. These are the best days of your life." (Honestly, would you want to do high school again?)

I'm sure you smiled when you read some of those examples; maybe you cringed at others. The point is that all parents have said things like this at some time or another. To add up to an invalidating environment, however, these messages must be pervasive, delivered over and over again. The invalidation has to somehow negate the private experience of the child. For example, in the "hungry" example above, if the child is experiencing a growling stomach, thoughts of food, and salivation, and believes she is hungry but then is told by older people that she is not, over time she will come to disbelieve her own experiences of hunger. Although eating disorders are thought to be a lot more complicated than this, this kind of invalidation surrounding hunger is one factor that can lead to disordered eating. So, the invalidation has to contradict the experiences of the child and must be prevalent and ongoing.

> *Remember, time is an important factor in the recipe for BPD. An environment becomes invalidating only when the invalidating messages are pervasive and delivered over and over.*

Before you read any further, I want to make one thing perfectly clear: Parents can contribute to an invalidating environment without being awful, abusive, insensitive people and without having anything but the best intentions for their child. I've met many people with BPD who were simply born to parents who are much less emotional than they are. Their parents meant well but just didn't know what their emotionally vulnerable child needed. They didn't understand that the child couldn't help being emotionally sensitive and reactive and that his or her emotions really tended to hang on, and so they couldn't help the child learn to regulate the emotions. This is particularly likely to be the case when any other children in the family resemble the parents in emotional temperament.

Also, although family of origin forms a big part of a child's environment, it's not the only part. A child could be strongly affected by an invalidating school environment—surrounded by rejecting peers or misguided by teachers who didn't know what he or she needed. Our entire Western society thrives on the idea that individuals should be self-reliant, autonomous, rational, logical, and in control of emotions at all times. To a child born with a highly charged emotional system, messages from all of these parts of the environment can be invalidating.

With these points in mind, then, let's talk about the kinds of invalidating environments your loved one might have been exposed to.

Where "Goodness of Fit" Is Missing

A few decades ago, Alexander Thomas and Stella Chess wrote extensively on "goodness of fit" in families. A family that has a good fit, from our standpoint, is one that can teach behaviors and model them for children. This requires that there be some similarity in the level of emotionality between the child and the caregivers, as mentioned briefly above. Sometimes a child who is extremely emotionally sensitive is born into a family of people who are substantially less emotional. The parents cannot show the child how to be good at being emotionally sensitive even if they are adept at regulating their own emotions.

I tell clients that for them this would be like being a swan born into a family full of ducks. The ducks cannot teach the swan how to be a swan; they can only teach her how to be a duck. Ducks aren't better than swans, and swans aren't better than ducks. They are just different. The problem is that the swan feels different, and if the ducks can't at least acknowledge that the swan is different, the act of learning how to be a duck, when you are a swan, is horribly invalidating.

An emotionally sensitive child born into a family of people who are less emotional may feel different from the beginning. Though the family may not realize that the child is different, or not know how to react even if they do know she is more emotional, they may still cope well with their own level of emotionality. However, they do not teach the more emotional child how to regulate more intense, long-lasting emotions. They're simply flabbergasted by them—or, worse, mortified by them, a message of unacceptability that they pass on to their child.

If you are the adult partner of someone with BPD, by the way, you may very well be a person who is able to validate your loved one in ways that his or her family of origin could not. It's been my informal observation that people with BPD often regulate themselves externally, meaning they depend to some extent on others to supply what they know they can't do for themselves. So many people with the disorder fall in love with compassionate, empathic individuals—*people who stand the best possible chance of using strategies such as the ones described in this book to preserve their relationship and live long and fulfilling lives together.*

The take-home message here, whether you're the parent or the partner of someone with BPD, is that invalidating environments are not environments that set out to destroy a child. There's no point in immersing yourself in guilt for what you were unable to do for your child or blaming your partner's family for causing all of the problems the two of you are struggling with today.

In subtle ways, a family of origin can negate the experience of the child or try to make the child into something that she cannot emotionally be. I once had a client who told me she had suffered no significant trauma. However, she really struggled with being very suicidal and impulsive, had a husband whom she did not love, and had little direction in her life. She was extremely well educated and intelligent. She said that her invalidation came in the form of her parents making her play the cello. At the time, I had a caseload (about 15) of people with BPD who had had devastating childhoods. I have to say that I too was invalidating to her because I couldn't get what she found so invalidating about playing the cello.

Finally, I just asked her what was so difficult about the cello. The client knew exactly what the problem was. She hated the way the cello looked and sounded. Children made fun of her for playing the cello and said she looked funny with that big instrument between her legs. The client did not like performing at all. When she told her parents this, they told her it didn't matter. She was going to play the cello because they had spent money for it and had decided she was going to be a cellist. The outcome was that this young woman believed her parents didn't pay attention to her, that her desires were not sufficient or valid.

As I grew to know this young woman, I realized that her entire life to date had been a continuation of having to "play the cello." She was forced by her parents, her husband, and her environment to do things she didn't want to do or like to do. She wanted to be a pharmacist; her parents, her husband, and her teachers told her she needed to go to medical school. She flunked out of medical school. She didn't want to marry the man who became her husband; her family told her she should marry him. Her experience was that no one listened to her, that her thoughts of what she wanted and needed were negated, and that she was incapable of making her own decisions. As she grew older, she was very sensitive to someone telling her to do things she did not want to do or did not think were wise. She felt panic at the thought of doing any kind of work that was observed by others. This caused difficulties in our relationship because I was constantly asking her to role play with me and do things that she did not want to do. However, she could not stop doing what others wanted because she did not believe she deserved to do so. So, she stayed in relationships and jobs that she hated and became hopeless and suicidal.

"Never Let Them See You Cry"

There are environments where people find it difficult to tolerate a lot of emotion and attempt to shut it down. This can happen for a variety of reasons. Maybe the parents were raised to find displays of emotion distasteful, and that attitude became distorted to include all emotional experience, not just emotional expression. Think of this environment as one in which a child comes home from school and is upset because she got a bad grade on a paper. She is told that she is overreacting and needs to just "suck it up" and come to dinner. There is no communication that her behavior is understandable. The sucking it up almost seems like some kind of magical tool that others have that the child does not. The result of this environment is that the child develops unrealistic problem-solving skills.

I once knew a teenager who was a beautiful child. She came from a family with a lot of money. Both of her parents were beautiful people, and her sister was a runway model. The teenager believed that she was the ugly one in the family. This perception was reinforced by her mother, who was constantly criticizing what she ate and how she looked, and lamenting that she did not look like her sister. The teenager decided that she would learn tennis, and she took lessons all summer. She was really enjoying tennis but was very anxious on the day of her first tennis match. Unfortunately, she lost that match miserably. She was very sad and pretty humiliated. As she walked off the court, she told her mother how awful she felt. Her mother responded by saying, "Honey, it would have been all right if you had just smiled." There was no communication about how hard it is to practice something all summer and then be disappointed by your performance and feel humiliated. In fact, what the girl learned was that all problems can be solved with a smile.

"You're Just Making It Up"

Another situation that arises from the invalidating environment is that the child's behaviors are considered unacceptable or "crazy." This is the child who is told that he doesn't know what he's talking about. Also, this child is criticized for the intensity of emotions. The child is often accused of overreacting and of behaving the way she behaves to "manipulate" people, to get things, like attention, or to get out of things, like going to physical education. The child does not learn what to do with emotions, just that she is a "bad person" for having them. This is the child who is at the theater with his parents and begins to wiggle. His parents tell him to hush. He wiggles more. His parents hush him louder. They tell him this is misbehavior and he needs to quit making a nuisance of himself. Finally, his mother drags him out into the lobby to scold him, only to have him throw up. He was wiggling because he was feeling nauseous.

This usually causes one of two things to happen: either the person becomes more emotional and out of control or the person begins to overcontrol emotions and shuts them down. This can lead to "dissociation," or the cutting off of emotion, described in Chapter 1. The person goes emotionally blank. Or the person can stuff the emotion down until it ultimately explodes, usually into a self-harm event (cutting or a suicide attempt) or an anger outburst.

Absent Parents

The invalidating environment can also be one in which parents are absent. This may be voluntary (a parent works all the time and is never home for the child) or forced (the parent is sent off to war). The reality is that children cannot learn to regulate emotion if there are no adults around to model behaviors. I had a client once who came to me asking about the development of BPD. She said she had never been abused and that she had a good relationship with her parents. However, she suffered from extreme loneliness and had many physical complaints and had been suicidal and anorexic for 10 years. The problem in the family was that her brother, who was 2 years younger, developed brain cancer as a young child. Her parents spent several years taking the boy to different hospitals. He had traumatic surgeries, and the parents spent weeks in hospitals. No one can fault the parents for doing what they had to do. The girl was at home with nannies and other family members who rotated caring for her. This young, very sensitive little girl learned that she wasn't as important as someone who was sick, and there was no consistent model of behavior to teach her what to do with all of the myriad emotions that arose naturally in growing up and as a result of having a terminally ill brother.

Sexual Abuse

Of course, the most invalidating of all environments is one where the child is being sexually molested. The adult treats the child in ways that the child knows, intuitively, are not right and then tells him that it is a secret or that he enjoys it. The child might tell the adult that it hurts or that he doesn't want to do it, but the adult does not respond and continues to molest him. There may even be threats of harm to the child or others. The child begins to stifle responses, telling himself that the adult knows more than he does, and begins to negate his own experience of reality.

It's important to know that not all people who develop BPD were sexually molested. Depending on the study that you read, 40–75% of people with BPD were sexually abused as children. Twenty-five to 75% were physically abused as children.

Even more devastating to the child is when he, as a child or an adult, tells family members or others about the abuse and is either ignored or accused of fabricating. I have seen this many times: the adult person with BPD decides to "come clean" and tell his family about who was sexually abusing him as a child. The family basically implodes, and the person is accused of lying, seeking attention, or trying to cause the family to split up. The consequence is even further invalidation. I think the reason this is so difficult is that when the abuse is occurring, and even afterward, the child often protects himself by thinking that his parents/family couldn't possibly have known what was going on, because if they had, they would have stopped it. Then, when the person realizes that he wouldn't have been believed, the devastation is complete. I have seen many people attempt suicide after this occurred.

Other Abuse and Criminal Behavior

Other invalidating environments can be ones where there is physical or emotional abuse or where a parent is abusing substances or involved in criminal behaviors. Often, in these situations, family members punish or trivialize the experiences of the child. This is the family that is constantly saying, "Quit that crying or I'll give you something to cry about." Just think about that statement for a minute. The child has an emotional reaction to a situation (maybe someone said something that hurt her feelings). Sadness wells up inside of her, and tears are the physiological expression of sadness, so they begin to well up in her eyes. Then the adult communicates that there was not a justifiable reason for the sadness. So the inner experience of the child is negated. Because the child is emotionally sensitive, she doesn't learn not to have emotions; she learns that she can't trust her own emotional experiences, that they are wrong. The effect is that she becomes more emotional, not less. And she will grow into someone who does not know her own emotions, cannot label them, tries to shut them down, and/or judges them as bad or wrong.

The Emotionally Sensitive Child Affects the Environment Too

So, it takes two things that come together to create BPD: an innate, biologically high level of emotions and an invalidating environment that punishes, trivializes, or ignores the inner experiences of the child and does not teach her how to regulate emotions. It is kind of a chicken-or-the-egg thing: it doesn't matter which came first. It's difficult to be the emotionally sensitive child, and it's difficult to be the family of the emotionally sensitive child. If you were in the family of origin of the person with BPD, I am sure you know what I mean: the level of emotion in the sensitive child also affects the environment.

Billy is in the grocery store with his mother and his sister. In the cereal aisle, Billy tells Mom that he wants a type of cereal that is full of sugar. Mom says no. Billy starts crying that he wants the cereal. Mom is embarrassed and starts shushing Billy. Billy cries louder. Mom finally grabs Billy and leaves the store. If you are the sister, your entire experience at the store just changed. Bewildered, you follow Billy and Mom from the store, wondering what became of the cart full of groceries. The shopping has ended. What happened was that there was a transaction between Mom and Billy. Billy's emotions affected Mom's emotions, which affected Billy's emotions. This happens repeatedly in families. The child and the environment are constantly affecting each other.

> - When an emotionally vulnerable child's inner experience is negated, she learns that she can't trust her emotions and grows into someone who doesn't understand them or what they're called, considers them bad or wrong, and either cries out louder and louder to be understood or does everything possible to suppress emotion.
> - Families can create an invalidating environment just by being emotionally different from the child and being unable to teach the child how to manage his own emotions.
> - Families are affected by the emotions of the child just as the child is affected by her emotions.

Now, think about what could happen next with Billy. What happens if Mom is mortified by Billy's crying and just wants him to stop, so she grabs the cereal that he wants and just shoves it at him? Billy quits crying, and they go on with their shopping. Billy has just had crying in the grocery store reinforced. Even though he is not aware of it, he is learning that escalating his emotional response results in his getting what he wants. This is how the child and the environment develop over time. The environment reacts to the emotions, and the emotions change the environment. If the emotionally sensitive child has the internal experience of feeling like a burn patient, to the family she can be like fingernails on a chalkboard. She becomes upset about something and the family naturally responds, which makes her upset, which makes the family respond and so on and so on.

*W*hat Now?

The question is: What do you do now? You have this person in your life, and you may even have some idea now of what contributed to the development of BPD in your loved one. However, she is still so easily upset with you. You think things are going well, and you get a phone call in the middle of the night telling you that she is going to kill herself because she knows you don't love her and she is a bad person who does not deserve to live. Or she comes home from work furious with her boss and cannot calm down. You keep trying to say helpful things, but they only make things worse.

I'll get into specifics about what you can do to have a better relationship with your loved one, and maybe even help him with his BPD symptoms, later in the book. But for now, let's look at how understanding the way people come by BPD lays the foundation for effective treatment and new ways of responding by those who love them.

Guidelines from the Biosocial Theory

The explanation of what creates BPD that you just read is called the *biosocial theory of borderline personality disorder*: your loved one came by this problem by virtue of innate emotional traits plus an environment that, intentionally or unintentionally, invalidated his or her childhood emotional experience. What you need to know about this theory right now is simply that it carves a direct route to the best treatment and new, beneficial ways of interacting with the person you care so much about.

Don't Try to Talk Your Loved One Out of Feeling the Way She Does

The first thing is to remember what you know about emotional sensitivity. Don't negate the cue. In other words, don't tell your loved one that she is overreacting or that she "shouldn't" be upset, even if you are doing so with the intention of helping her feel better. With an emotional regulation system that is hypersensitive, she probably "should" be upset. Placating her will only make things worse. Don't tell her that she should not be so upset, that things are not as bad as they seem. You are then challenging the intensity of her emotional reaction. What will this do? Escalate the reaction.

Don't Remake Your World to Accommodate Your Loved One's Emotional "Fragility"

When you care about someone with BPD, you can end up feeling severely punished by her high level of emotion. You often try to respond in helpful ways when she is upset about something, and it backfires.

Your loved one becomes more upset or becomes upset with you. Over time, you may find yourself so tired and afraid of the emotion that you try to create a world that does not upset your loved one. I know this is going to sound cavalier, but don't do it. It is imperative not to treat the person with BPD like she is fragile when she's not or try to create a world that is not upsetting, especially if she is in DBT. The only way the person with BPD is going to survive is to learn how to live in this world, not an artificial world that is designed to keep her emotion under control. However, the balance is that you may need to have some time where you focus on caring for your own emotions. This may mean distancing yourself for a period of time (usually an hour or so is long enough to let emotions simmer down) while waiting for the long-lasting emotions of your loved one to cool.

Understand the Tasks of Emotional Regulation That Your Loved One Needs to Be Able to Perform

Now you know a lot about how your loved one got where he or she is today. Before we move on to how you can interact in ways that will serve you and your relationship well, it will help if you understand exactly what emotional regulation means and what your loved one will have to learn to do to lead a fulfilling life and keep the relationships so important to her. To regulate emotion, we all need to be able to:

- **Reorient attention**—do something that is not related to what is upsetting us (distract ourselves).
- **Up-regulate or down-regulate our physiological arousal.** Emotions either increase our physiological arousal, as does anger, which causes all of our internal systems to crank up, or decrease our physiological arousal, like sadness, which causes all of our internal systems to slow down. Emotion regulation requires that we be able to bring down our arousal when cranked up (angry, fearful, disgusted) and bring up our arousal when low (sadness, shame).
- **Stop ourselves from doing whatever it is our emotion and mood tell us to do.** Going with our mood is called "mood dependent behavior," implying that we're not in charge; our moods are.
- **Have a life with goals in it that are independent of emotion** that we can move toward when the going gets rough, like volunteering, or working toward a new job.

So, let's go back to the scenario where your loved one comes home furious at her boss and can't seem to calm down about having had a very bad day and see how you could handle it with your new understanding:

1. Ask what has happened and listen without contradicting, judging, and making comments about the intensity of her reaction.
2. Then find something about what she has said that you can acknowledge made sense. This could be specific: "I would be angry if I felt criticized by my boss, too." Or it could be more general: "It sounds like you had a really bad day. I understand that you may need some time to decompress."
3. Then ask if you can help by providing some distraction—take her out to dinner, play a game, or turn on her favorite movie. Do something that does not involve the cue for her emotion, meaning you should not rehash what happened. You can help her do something to soothe her nerves (if her upset is anger or fear, not sadness), like take a warm bath, listen to calming music, or, believe it or not, put her face in very cold water (it makes the body's arousal systems drop dramatically and quickly). You can help her avoid going with whatever her emotion is making her want to do: pick up the phone and call someone, hit something, and so forth. You can get her talking about her long-term goals (hopefully she has some, because now would not be the time to discuss establishing some).

But what if your loved one is not in a place where she will allow herself to be helped by you and you cannot suggest anything she will find helpful? If you do suggest something, will she find it invalidating because you're treating her like she can't figure things out herself? If possible, let her be. Remember that emotionally sensitive people have emotions that last longer than those of others. But even if her emotional reaction seems interminable, it will end if no more cues come up. All you can do in those moments is try not to invalidate her further by communicating that she should be over it, that she is overreacting, or that she is out of line.

If you can't seem to help your loved one calm down, and you don't even really have any idea what's upsetting her, the key to an appropriate response is what we call *assessment*: Ask questions about her internal experiences and then listen to the answer without filtering or judging what your loved one is saying. With my patient who felt like her whole life was characterized by being forced to play the cello, I began with a simple question: "I've noticed that whenever I ask you to practice something in here you get really emotional. Can you tell me what happens?"

Know That Change Will Be Painful for Your Loved One

Think of the intense emotionality of BPD as being like having severe burns. Despite your burns being covered in salve and mesh, your wounds are exposed to the world. Not only is any movement of your own excruciating, but even the force of the air when hospital workers walk by causes you pain, and that pain lasts for an interminable period of time. Such is the emotional situation of those with BPD. They have emotional responses that are huge and last a long, long time.

The problem with the burn patient, of course, is that the most agonizing thing that happens to them is the treatment provided. Everything that is ultimately going to help them heal causes the person with burns exquisite pain. This, unfortunately, is true with people with BPD. The treatments that are most effective often cause them pain for a sustained period of time. DBT asks people to give up the means by which they've been soothing their pain, possibly for years—whether it's alcohol or drugs, cutting or suicide attempts, unprotected sex or lashing out at loved ones. In return, DBT gives them the skills they need to be able to perform the tasks of emotional regulation, but it can be a long haul, during which the person has to experience the emotions that have caused her so much pain. Fortunately, DBT gives people lots of methods for distracting themselves that are healthy and lots of options that will head off harmful impulsive behavior. But I can't tell you that it will be easy. I can tell you that things will get better if you use the ideas offered in this book, and they may get better faster if your loved one can consult a qualified DBT therapist; see Chapter 13 for more information.

I've given you a lot to think about in this chapter, so I want to review it for a moment. First, we use a biosocial theory of the development of BPD. This means that people with BPD are born with a biological emotional vulnerability. They have big emotions that occur often and easily, and last a long time. However, not everyone who is emotionally vulnerable grows up to have BPD. The second ingredient that is required is the invalidating environment. The invalidating environment is one where the private (and public) experiences of the child are punished, treated as inaccurate, ignored, or negated, and/or the child is not taught how to regulate emotions. To regulate emotions, all people need to be able to (1) do things that are not about what is causing the emotion, (2) regulate their bodies down (when the emotion increases their physiological arousal) or up (when the emotion decreases their arousal), (3) not engage in behavior that is about the current mood or emotion (i.e., not go with the emotion), and (4) have a life that involves goals independent of the emotion so that in the moment they can focus on them. Finally, if your loved one is emotionally upset, remember the biosocial theory is the answer to why he is responding as he is.

In a nutshell, here are some suggestions for things to do that incorporate the biosocial theory:

1. Assess: ask what has happened.
2. Listen actively; don't contradict, judge, or say your loved one is overreacting.
3. Validate: find something in what happened that makes sense and is understandable, that you can relate to; say what that it is.
4. Ask if you can help, not to solve the problem but to get through the moment.
5. If your loved one says no, give him or her space and remember the emotions of emotionally vulnerable people last longer.

This sounds simple but obviously is not always easy to carry out in the heat of the moment; I'll give you a step-by-step process, with plenty of illustrations, for deciding exactly how to respond to your loved one in a way that will help you both in Chapter 4. Throughout this book, I will give you more suggestions for things to do, but the beginnings are always the same: assess (ask objective questions), listen to the answer, and validate. If you start with this, many times your loved one's emotions will begin to subside a little, just from the experience of having someone listen without invalidating. Chapter 3 will show you how validation works in more detail.

The Hidden Power of Validation

What happens when you do something nice for the person you love who has BPD? One woman I know kept trying to give her daughter what she needed to succeed in the workplace because the young woman was so convinced that keeping a good job would solve all the other problems in her life. At different times the mother provided college tuition, bought her a presentable wardrobe, offered to drive her to work, and attempted to coach her daughter on how to get along with coworkers. But every time she made these generous gestures, her daughter would burst into tears, attack her with angry accusations, or sink into a silent depression. Eventually the mother stopped trying.

A man I know tried over and over to get his sister help for substance abuse, introduced her to people he thought would be more supportive friends than the ones she met in bars, and offered to go to therapy sessions with her if it would make the experience easier. She either ignored his offers or said, "Sure, thanks," and then never followed through. After a couple years the brother stopped asking.

Another man I know has been acting as his wife's "keeper" for years. He arranges social events so that people who "upset" her won't be there. He leaves work to go home and "talk her down" when she can't handle her own distress. He handles all their financial affairs so she doesn't have to worry about the fact that she can't hold down a job that would pay for her impulsive purchases. His wife thanks him profusely every time he paves the way or bails her out, so he figures he's on the right track and seems to think of new ways to "help" each week.

Responses Matter—Sometimes a Lot More Than We Think

There is a basic fact of human behavior: we are all affected by principles of reinforcement, extinction, and punishment. In plain English, this means that if you try to do kind things for your loved one and she responds negatively, you will eventually be deterred from doing kind things (punishment). You will actually avoid doing kind things for her to spare yourself her reactions. It also means that if you try to help and she ignores your attempts, you will eventually stop trying to help (extinction: she doesn't react in a way that is reinforcing, which thereby extinguishes your helping behavior). You may still want to help her, but your helping behaviors will just stop. If you intervene and try to arrange everything in the world so that your loved one does not get upset, and she heaps gratitude on you (assuming you're motivated by thanks), you will keep intervening and may in fact increase your interventions (reinforcement).

The three people I just described stopped doing what they were doing or kept doing it *because of the reaction they got.* The reactions of their loved ones with BPD didn't necessarily make sense, and weren't necessarily intended to hurt the people who were trying so hard to help them. But those reactions couldn't help evoking reactions of their own: a mother and a brother ceased their well-intended attempts to help, and a husband inadvertently encouraged his wife to stay captive to her runaway emotions rather than learning to master them. The inescapable lesson here is that when we deal with others, we really have to pay attention to our responses.

The reality is that the behaviors you encounter from your loved one with BPD can be punishing. Not that your loved one is *trying* to punish you, but the emotional reactions of people with BPD can make us feel despondent, angry, hopeless, and helpless, among other emotions. Naturally, being human beings, we can react to those emotions. Animals stop engaging in behaviors that are punished. Think of rats in a maze. They hit a lever to get food. But what if they hit the lever for the food and get an electric shock? They will stop eating and will eventually die because they are avoiding the punishment of the electric shock. This happens in relationships. If our behavior in a relationship is punished, we will quit the behavior. We react. Then the person with

BPD reacts to our reactions. I'm sure you see where this is going, because you've been there so many times before.

We need a way to start at the beginning and manage the cascade of responses. The best way to do so is to defuse some of the emotionality that presents itself in our interactions with our loved ones. This means regulating our own emotions but also helping to bring down emotion in our loved ones, who are so subject to high emotion. If we don't accomplish this, our interactions are unlikely to go where we want them to go.

People cannot pay attention well or participate in conversations when they are emotionally dysregulated.

Interrupting the usual cascade of responses means not only regulating your own emotion but also helping the person with BPD do the same.

Here's how things go awry: Something happens, and the emotions of the person with BPD immediately start firing. In emotionally sensitive people, like those with BPD, there is not only the sense of the emotion itself, but also the sense of being emotionally out of control. It's a double whammy. The actual emotion is compounded by the experience of being out of control—even when the emotions are "normal" in their intensity and their occurrence. Once the person feels out of control, she will usually either attack verbally or physically, with some harm to herself or you, or withdraw, either by physically leaving the situation (often slamming the door behind her) or by dissociating (what appears to be "zoning out"). And, of course, when this happens, your relationship suffers and, if there was a problem that needed to be solved, nothing happens to solve it.

The emotions of people with BPD are aversive because they cause us to have more emotion, they aren't predictable, or they just don't make sense to us. Think about your loved one. Can you determine how he experiences emotions? Do his emotions happen in ways that you don't often understand, such as arising in response to something you would not have emotions about or lasting for long periods of time? It might be helpful to write down some of what you're noticing about your loved one's emotions right now. Here's an example of what I wrote down about a client:

1. She is easily hurt by my responses. I think I am being helpful, and she thinks I am being critical.
2. She often leaves sessions and seems like she is okay emotionally.

Then she calls a few hours (or days) later to tell me that she hates me because I am mean. When I ask what I did, I normally don't even remember what she reports I said, and when we listen to our session tape, often I did not say what she heard.

3. If I miss something (like she is having an emotion that I don't notice), she thinks I don't care about her and becomes despondent.

4. She stays upset with me for weeks, independent of how hard I try to make things right between us.

5. She interprets my responses to her as meaning she is "stupid, worthless, a bad person," and so forth.

If I didn't have ways to defuse emotions or somehow change the tenor of them at the beginning of our interactions, what do you think could happen between me and this client? We could end up in huge arguments. I could conclude that this person was just "crazy" and start treating her as if she were hopeless. I could end up resenting all the effort I put in and the lack of gratitude that I got in return. I could let our relationship fizzle out on its own, relieved when I didn't hear from her because she was mad at me. I could start putting all kinds of limits on our relationship to protect my own right to privacy and peace that would feel like rejection to her. I might end up giving up on this client. You too could end up giving up on the relationship you have with someone who has BPD.

$\mathcal{V}$alidation Reduces Emotional Intensity

I know you're not prepared to give up on your relationship at this time, and this is why I'm devoting a whole chapter to validation. It's a response you can use in any interaction with your loved one, and you'll find it has power beyond anything you can imagine to bring down emotion to a more manageable level and put your encounter on a more fruitful course. It is at the very center of any helpful response to a person with BPD.

Sometimes, just telling another person about a situation and your emotions can make you feel more emotional. Just think of times when some injustice has been done to you, and maybe your fury had calmed a bit until you got home and had a chance to recount the incident to a family member. All of a sudden you can find yourself every bit as angry as you were when it happened. Just the act of talking about it can cause your emotions to go up.

Now picture your family member saying "I understand what you're saying" or "I can see where you're coming from" or "Of course you feel that way. Anyone would." When you get that response, don't you physically feel your emotion settling down a little? But what if the other person says "You shouldn't feel that way" or somehow dismisses what you say? What happens to your emotion? It goes up, and your ability to listen to the other person goes down.

> *Validation helps to bring down emotions and make them more manageable for everyone, not just the person with BPD.*

*V*alidation Authenticates Some Part of a Person's Internal Experience

Validation is a concept that is prevalent in our culture. If you park in a garage connected to a restaurant, the garage attendant will often give you a ticket and tell you to have it "validated" at the restaurant for a reduction in the parking fees. When a restaurant employee stamps the ticket, he's saying that you did, in fact, go to the restaurant. The validated ticket corroborates your claim that you parked in the garage to use the restaurant's facilities. This is basically the function of DBT validation: it authenticates some aspect of the experience of another person.

There is a professor named Bill Swann at the University of Texas who researches how people interact. His theory is that we all have what he calls "self-constructs." Self-constructs are how we see ourselves. There are some basic self-constructs: who we are, where we are heading in our lives, what is hard for us, what is easy for us. People with BPD often have self-constructs of being out of control, having a lot of emotional pain, not being able to tolerate emotional pain, not being able to do things that others can do, not having a sense of who they are—essentially a representation of the five areas of dysregulation discussed in Chapter 1. Even if our self-constructs are negative, it's human nature for us to look for people to verify or validate them. We gravitate toward people who do not challenge our beliefs about ourselves. I am a person with fair skin and freckles. However, because I spent most of my time on the beach when I was a child, and because the other members of my family are not as fair, I thought I had olive skin. When I was 16, a lifeguard told me that I needed sunscreen because I was fair. Not only was I incensed, but I went around Hawaii for a week asking people if they thought I had fair skin. I was looking for anyone who believed I had olive skin so that I could hang out on the beach with them. I was looking for validation of my self-construct of having olive skin. Not only that, but I was so dysregulated and distraught about being told I was fair skinned that the entire trip to Hawaii was ruined and I am sure I made my family miserable.

A self-construct does not have to be "true" or "real." It is a belief about who we are and how we experience the world. So, if your loved one has an identity that includes thinking that she is worthless and undeserving of love and you are constantly (out of love, of course) telling her that she is wrong, that she is not worthless and undeserving of love, she will become more emotional around you and may well turn to her relationship with the violent drug addict who actually treats her like she's not worth anything and sometimes tells her outright that she has no value. This is not some attempt by the person you love to self-destruct. She is gravitating toward people whose manner of treating her is consistent with her own sense of who she is, where she is, and what she is all about.

This, of course, creates a kind of "catch-22" for those of us who love people with BPD. We want to assure our loved ones that they can be okay, that they can get control, that they do have meaning, but in the moment just saying those things can trigger a whole new wave of emotions.

Sometimes in our society we use the term *validate* to mean "agree." What I mean by *validation* is a little different: I mean finding one (sometimes very small) piece of a behavior (as a behaviorist I include thoughts, feelings, and/or actions in the term *behavior*) that is authentically understandable to you and communicating to the other person that it is understandable. You don't even necessarily have to agree with the behavior; you just have to be able to say honestly that you find it understandable. If it's not understandable to you, you don't validate it. That would be validating the invalid and can often be dangerous—it might mean reinforcing, through your own reaction, a behavior that is clearly harmful.

Finding something to validate can be really difficult. Consider a person who weighs 70 pounds and says she's fat. It probably is true that she has a self-construct of being a fat person. However, to agree with her that she is fat would be validating the invalid. Fortunately, there are things that we can validate. We all have had days when, independent of our weight, we *feel* fat, or we ate too much last night and are worried that we're gaining weight. Vocalizing these aspects—"I know you feel fat" or "Being bloated stinks" or "I can understand that you're worried about gaining weight even when you know you need to do so"—is validation. It's the communication that *some* of what the person says makes sense and is understandable to us.

> • *Validation is not the same thing as agreement (though it can be).*
> • *We never validate the invalid.*

Now think about what I just said about validation and what I said earlier about self-constructs. If you challenge people's self-constructs, they can become so dysregulated that they cannot hear anything else you say. I recently was training a group of therapists to conduct DBT. One group came into the training with DBT in their company name. They absolutely believed that they were providing the treatment (self-construct). I began consulting with them by saying, "This is not DBT." Because I had said they were not who they thought they were, they were so dysregulated that they could not process any of the information I wanted to give them. I had to back up and say, "I know you believe you are doing DBT and you want to do it." Then I had to ensure them that there were pieces of DBT in what they were doing. Their emotions calmed, and they could listen to the feedback that I gave. You may not agree with your loved one's self-constructs of being worthless and undeserving of love, but these are her reality. What would happen if you responded to her by saying, "You are not worthless and you do deserve love," which is arguing against her self-constructs? She would probably get more upset. You care about her and don't want to say "You're right. You're worthless and don't deserve love." Using validation, you would begin by saying, "Look, I know that you see yourself as worthless and undeserving. The fact is, you have done some things that have made you feel that way, and I know that your mistakes in life have made you feel bad about yourself. This is what I know about you, though ... " Here you get to say all of the things that you really want to say about how she is a basically decent human being, everyone deserves love, and so forth. Do you see that first you'd be validating her experience of herself and then moving on to say what you wanted to say? The validation is like the spoonful of sugar that helps the medicine go down. It communicates understanding and acknowledgment of the person's experience in a way that keeps emotional arousal down and allows for the rest of the statement. Some of people's self-constructs can change over time and with experience. Hopefully, as your loved one builds a life with different behaviors, her beliefs about her worthlessness will change.

*W*hat *Not* to Try Instead of Validation

There are some basic mistakes that we all make when people are emotional.

• *Don't tell your loved one to calm down.* Seriously, have you ever seen that work? When you tell someone to calm down, you are invalidating the person's upset, and emotions go up, not down.

• *Don't try to solve the problem before you have a clear picture of it and are sure your loved one wants you to solve it.* Another error is that we try to solve the problem. Many of us are good problem solvers, and the minute someone begins to tell us of something that is going on in her life, we see solutions and begin to offer our great ideas. Then the person just gets more upset. I know this used to happen with my husband and me. I would tell him about something that was going on, and I really just wanted him to listen and tell me that I was not mistaken in my response. As I would begin to tell him what was happening, he would say, "What you need to do is ... " and "I would just tell that person ... " I would feel the emotions building inside of me—mostly frustration—and have the sense of not being understood. Then I would be upset not only about the situation that I was telling him about but also with him for not listening. Validation requires listening without first moving to solve the problem.

> It is imperative when you validate someone that you be genuine and real in what you say.

• *Don't say you understand when you don't.* Sometimes people try to validate, and what they say or do comes out as placating and condescending. Have you ever had someone say to you "I know what you mean," which only made you think, "You do not; you have *no* idea what I mean"? Again, emotions rise.

How to Validate

Let me repeat a really critical point here: Validation does not have to mean agreeing with the other person. Often we *don't* agree with what the person with BPD is doing. For example, we do not agree with his going out to bars, getting drunk, picking up men, and having unprotected sex because he had an argument with his boss. But if your loved one shows up at your house afterward and you immediately tell him what his mistakes were and how unsafe his behavior was and what a problem his coping method is, you will not be heard and your loved one will become even more out of control. The key is timing. When you find something valid to validate, you can postpone your own agenda of pointing out where your loved one needs to make changes to protect himself and others, and by the time you get to that, he just might hear you.

Of course holding back to find the perfect timing is not easy, especially when emotions are heating up. That's why DBT breaks validation into six levels that can keep you focused on controlling your own response even when the person with BPD seems and feels out of control.

The Six Levels of Validation (from Marsha Linehan)

Before I begin teaching you the levels of validation and how to do them, I want to be clear. I am going to spend most of my time telling you how to validate the person with BPD, but validating yourself and other people who love the person with BPD is also important. In fact, when anyone is dysregulated, it is a good idea to validate the person before you do anything else. Even if your partner is not the person in your life with BPD, if he comes home distressed about something that happened at work, validation has been shown as a sure way to keep conflict down. Self-validation is an important part of regulating your own emotions, so practice validating your own experiences as well those of your loved one. I'll talk more about self-validation at the end of the chapter.

Level 1: Stay Awake

Validating a person who is emotionally aroused is a skill. It is pretty easy to validate someone who is not upset. All you really have to do is listen and nod. When the person is upset, listening and nodding might work. Have you had that work for you? You were distressed about something and you told someone. Maybe the other person didn't have any brilliant ideas, but the fact that he just sat, gave you time, and listened, seemingly objectively, made your emotions quiet somewhat. This is what we call the first level of validation, *staying awake*.

Staying awake requires that you pay attention and ask objective, probing questions—basically that you demonstrate that you're paying attention to the person who is talking. Lean forward, nod your head, ask questions that show you are paying attention.

A big piece of staying awake (and all levels of validation, actually) is not being judgmental about what the other person is saying to you. Let's go back to the man who gets drunk and has sex with men he doesn't know. He comes to you—his mother, his friend, his father—whoever you are. He looks terrible, hung over, eyes red and swollen. He is obviously distraught and begins to tell you about last night. It would be somewhat natural to find the thought "What a stupid, careless thing to do" going through your mind. But it's important not to entertain such judgments when you find them popping into your head, because people with BPD are very sensitive to criticism and typically can see the changes on our faces that reflect judgmental thoughts.

How do you disengage from judgmental thoughts? The first step is to concentrate on what the other person is saying. If you're paying complete attention (we call it being mindful), you will not be able to participate in judging. The second step is to stay focused on the facts of the situation and not allow yourself to engage in opinion forming or evaluating. Mind you, this is a very difficult skill to master. Our minds seem to rush to judgment, and judgments come out of our mouths often without our even thinking about them. Practice being nonjudgmental in times that are not crisis times. Notice the thoughts that go through your mind. Are they facts or evaluations? Start taking words like *good*, *bad*, *right*, *wrong*, *fair*, and *unfair* out of your vocabulary. Let go of extreme words like *always*, *never*, *no one*, and *everyone*. These are the beginnings of taking a nonjudgmental stance. Realize, also, that we sometimes judge without meaning to do so. Don't get judgmental of the judgments of yourself. Let go of judgments and pay very close attention to the person, communicating that you're listening.

Level 2: Accurate Reflection

Accurate reflection requires you to communicate that you've heard the person accurately. Sometimes people will just repeat, verbatim, what the other person has said. Therapists learn to do this in graduate school. The person who's playing the role of the client says, "It was really hard for me, and I struggled with it a lot." The person who's learning to be a therapist responds, "What I hear you saying is that it was hard for you and you struggled with it a lot." Now, this simple technique has a place with someone who is terribly upset or who is very concrete in his thinking. But I have to tell you, when someone does it to me, it almost becomes invalidating. I feel like I'm in the room with a parrot.

Nevertheless, you can use this level of validation when accuracy is part of the validation. Just make sure you change the wording around so that the person realizes you get the gist of what he is saying. Let's say he says, "I cannot believe that I went out and got wasted last night. I'm worried about what can happen next." You can then say something like "Hmm, you're really concerned about the consequences of last night and feel bad about getting wasted." Whether you restate verbatim or restate the gist, the result is that you communicate to a person who largely feels that his responses to the world are illogical and don't make sense that what he is experiencing is universal enough for you to "get it."

Level 3: Stating the Unarticulated

I call this mind reading. Mind reading requires that you create a little hypothesis about what the person is not telling you. It is usually best to present it in question form, or ask if it is accurate, especially when the person is highly dysregulated. So, with the example above, you could say, "I bet you're worried about an STD from last night. Is that right?" or "You must really be beating up on yourself for doing something you had sworn not to do again, huh?" The key to mind reading is that you have

> *The levels of validation are fluid and can often be used with each other.*

to be willing to be wrong. The person may respond, "No, I'm really not worried about STDs at all. I know people who have had relationships with that guy, and he's fine." The best response in this case is to follow up with a question that is more like Level 1 (staying awake): "Okay. So, what is it here that really has you worried? What are those consequences that you're talking about?"

The next two levels of validation are very powerful. They involve normalizing the person's responses.

Level 4: Validating in Terms of Personal History or Biology

Because in any one moment we are the sum total of every moment in our lives, on some level, our behavior makes sense. It may not be functional or make sense in the context of our larger society, but it makes sense given who we are and what has happened in our lives. For example, I know someone whose home burned down during a storm when she was about five. Her family lost everything in the fire. She lives in a place that is given to powerful summer storms with many lightning strikes. When there is lightning, she becomes very anxious and often sits in a closet until the storm is over. However, her profession requires that she care for others during storms, so in terms of the present, hiding in closets is an invalid behavior. Using Level 4 validation, I might say something like "I really understand why you want to hide in closets during storms. Your house burned down in a storm. It makes perfect sense that seeing lightning causes you to get really anxious. It's a part of your personal history." I could then move into how her behavior (hiding in the closet) is no longer helpful, but first I would want to point out my understanding that having a history with such loss and fear affects who she is at this moment.

Another Level 4 validation is validation in terms of a person's own biology. Our physiology, our physical problems, how our body reacts to the world affect our behavioral responses to the world. For example, people with attention-deficit/hyperactivity disorder (ADHD) have a hard time paying attention throughout a 4-hour class. People with disc problems in their backs have a difficult time sitting through a 4-hour class. Both of these examples are biological in nature. The key in using this type of validation is to find a way that the person's behavior makes sense without pathologizing the person or making it sound as if he is somehow defective. Remember the person who went to the bar? I could say to him: "I understand why you went to that bar. When you've had a bad day, your craving for alcohol goes way up. That's what started the whole thing." Notice I'm not saying that going to the bar was a good idea or that he should have gone to the bar. I have enough knowledge of the effects of alcohol on physiological craving that I can understand why one thing led to another. I could go further in the conversation. I could address the concerns about what happened later: "Alcohol really does disinhibit you, so it probably does happen that you leave bars with people when you drink."

Level 5: Normalizing

Level 5 is so important because it communicates that others (without BPD) would have the same response. People with BPD have the ongoing experience of being different—outsiders in their own worlds. When you normalize you find a way to communicate that what is going on for the person with BPD is the experience of being human, that anyone in the same situation would feel the same way. This is very powerful. Some key phrases that can be used are:

> "We all have moments when we feel that way."
> "Of course you think that; anyone would in your situation."
> "I would feel that way, too."
> "You know that is such a normal reaction."
> "It makes sense that you did that. We all have those moments."

Let's compare this to Level 4 for the person who had a problem with storms. I validated the woman's fear of storms based on personal history by saying "I really understand why you want to hide in closets during storms. Your house burned down in a storm. It is makes perfect sense that seeing lightning causes you to get really anxious. It's a part of your personal history." If I were to normalize her behavior, I would say something like "Listen, storms are scary. Most people want to do something to get away from the lightning and the thunder when they are happening." Notice that I am not saying that this is a response that is particular to her. It is a perfectly normal reaction to be afraid of storms.

The same can be done for the biology examples in Level 4. For the person who has ADHD, instead of saying "People with ADHD have a hard time paying attention during a 4-hour class," at Level 5 validation I would say something like "It's hard to pay attention to the same topic for 4 hours at a time." For the person with the back problems, instead of saying " People with disc problems in their backs have a difficult time sitting through a 4-hour class," I would say, "These chairs are hard on your back." See the difference? One is about the person in particular; the second is about humans in general.

Sometimes there is no way to normalize behavior. I can't really say to someone, "People get suicidal when their feelings get hurt" or "We all feel like cutting when we have had a really stressful day." **Don't normalize behavior that is not normal—that's validating the invalid.** If the person with BPD understands that his behavior is invalid, trying to normalize it will only send emotions soaring. In those cases, it's better to go for Level 4 validation: "I know that you have suicidal thoughts when you have days like today. It's your immediate response" or "I understand that when you've had a bad day you just want to do something to feel better, and cutting has been that thing for you."

Level 6: Radical Genuineness

The key to all of validation is to be genuine. Sometimes when I hear people trying to validate, they're using all the right words, but their tone of voice sounds parental or patronizing. Level 6 validation is exactly what the words say: Be radically genuine with your loved one with BPD.

There's no doubt that this can be really hard. It's difficult to be yourself with a ticking time bomb. The idea is not to treat your loved one any differently than you would any one in any other circumstance. Many times, especially in the mental health field, we treat people like they are more fragile than they really are. To be radically genuine is to ensure that you do not "fragilize," condescend, or talk down to the person you are trying to validate.

This can be done directly with words or by your manner. For example, if a friend of mine calls and says she has had the worst day of her life—she is about to lose her job, she came home to find the kids had written all over her walls, and she is sure her husband is having an affair—I say, "Oh my gosh. How terrible. What can I do?" I don't ask her if she needs to go to an emergency room. I don't talk to her like she's a child. She has my attention and my sympathy, and I am treating her like a fully capable person.

I once had a client who was a very small person—about 4 feet, 11 inches tall. She was married to a man who was very tall, and her psychiatrist was a very large ex–football player. On several occasions, I watched these two men (with her best interests at heart to be sure) talk to her in a "baby voice" when she was upset. I never heard the men talk to a larger person in that tone of voice. In those moments, they were fragilizing my client. When they talked with her in these childlike voices, she did not get any more regulated. As a matter of fact, on the occasions that I witnessed the interactions, my client became more upset when the men were talking to her.

Level 6 validation, in a nutshell, is talking to your loved one like you would anyone else. The problem, of course, is that often your loved one does not seem to be (or really is not) as capable as others in your life. You may have a history of having had to "caretake" your loved one because of life circumstances. Or, it may be very easy to be paternal with your loved one because you are, in fact, the parent. However, remember that there are several really good reasons for changing your responses. Number one, my guess is that they haven't worked. Number two, the reason for validation is to dampen emotional arousal. Number three, there is really good evidence that people will act as you expect them to act. Thus, if you treat a person as fragile, she will be fragile. If you treat a person as competent, she will become competent.

Putting the Levels of Validation Together

Now let's put the beginning scenario together. We are going to call our loved one with BPD Ray. Ray calls you up in the morning. He is really upset; his voice is loud, and he sounds like he's on the verge of tears.

> RAY: I cannot believe what I did last night. I had a bad day. Bob and I are having really bad problems. I couldn't go home, so I went to the bar. [increasing dysregulation].
>
> YOU: Okay, Ray. You and Bob were in a bad place, and so you went to the bar and not home [Level 2]. Tell me what happened [Level 1].
>
> RAY: (louder) I'm telling you what happened. I got wasted and went home with someone I didn't know. I blacked out and don't remember what happened.
>
> YOU: Man, this is bad [Level 5]. You're worried about what you did last night, right [Level 3]? Are you worried about STDs or about what Bob thinks? I'd probably be worried about both [Level 5].

RAY: I don't want to talk about it anymore. It's pissing me off even talking about it.

YOU: I'm sure it's hard to talk about [Level 5]. I bet you have a lot of emotions right now [Level 3]. I know people have been hard on you before, and it's making it difficult for you to talk to me [Level 4]. Are you sure you don't want my help?

Validating Yourself and Others

We all need validation when distressed. Family members of people with BPD probably need more validation from each other than other family members. There are several groups of scientists who are studying validation in relationships, and they are finding that the art of validation makes all relationships function better. To validate other family members who don't have BPD, follow the same six levels of validation.

Also validate yourself, especially in the context of your loved one with BPD. When you recognize that you're becoming dysregulated, the first three levels (staying awake, accurate reflection, and mind reading) won't work and would be very artificial. However, you can apply Levels 4 and 5 to yourself. Look at your response and identify how your behavior makes sense given your history, your biology, or the current circumstances. Saying to yourself, "You are upset with him because you care about him. That's what parents do" is an example of normalizing your behavior. Taking the care to do this will allow your emotions to stay more regulated.

Practicing Validation

There are different ways to validate. You can validate a person's:

Thoughts: "I can see why you're worried about that. It's definitely a concern."

Emotions: "Of course you're sad about the breakup. It's devastating."

Actions: "I understand why you walked away from him instead of standing and arguing."

Point of view: "Of course you don't have to talk about that now."
Abilities: "I know you can do this. You absolutely have it in you."

To help you learn to recognize the need to validate, think of recent experiences with your loved one. Focus on an interaction where his or her emotional arousal increased and validation may have brought down the emotion.

In each blank, describe enough of the situation to remind you what the occasion was and then write a statement for each type of validation that you could have used in the situation.

Describe the situation. _____

_____

_____

_____

How did I know that my loved one's arousal was increasing? _____

_____

_____

_____

Examples of validation. I could say:

Thoughts: _____

_____

_____

Emotions: _____

_____

_____

Actions: _____

_____

_____

Point of view: _____

_____

_____

Abilities: _____

_____

_____

_____

*V*alidation in Action

When you respond differently to borderline behavior, your loved one reacts differently too, and these typical behavior patterns are much less likely to spiral into the crisis-generating, destructive, and self-destructive behaviors that can burn you out. Validation is one key part of reacting differently to keep emotions from escalating, and practicing using the preceding exercise is one way to make it a nearly automatic response. But validation is not the only tool you have at your disposal.

At the end of Chapter 2, I listed several things you can do to keep interactions with your loved one from disintegrating in a storm of emotion. In Chapter 4 I'll elaborate on those simple steps. Together, they can help you feel like finally there *is* something you can do when you get yet another distress call from your sister at 2:00 A.M. or your son shows up unannounced to demand that you get him out of the latest mess he's gotten himself into. These new ways of responding are based on everything you've just read about the five areas of dysregulation in BPD and are effective not only in crisis situations but also when you want to have a productive conversation about some long-standing issue without renegade emotions throwing up a brick wall.

Five Steps to Balanced Responses and Better Outcomes

By now I hope you've gained an understanding of what's behind the behaviors often seen in BPD and why it's so important to respond differently to them than you may have previously. If you read Chapter 3, you have an idea of why validation is so critical to heading off emotional dysregulation. But translating understanding into action is no easy feat, especially when you feel depleted by your helplessness to get your loved one to change. Many people who love someone with BPD reach a point where they feel like they just can't take another 2:00 A.M. distress call or one more unpleasant surprise. They can't bear to watch their loved one experience so much pain over and over. What are they supposed to do?

I tell those who love someone with BPD that understanding where borderline behaviors come from really does make a difference. But realistically, it takes time for a new understanding to produce change. That's why I've come up with five simple steps that you can use right now, to make a difference right now, whenever you find yourself overwhelmed by a crisis or want to keep a conversation on a productive track. These are steps that you can easily commit to memory, that you can rehearse until they're second nature, and that you can then pull out anytime emotion threatens to steal the show. At the end of the day, you can only change your own behavior—your responses to your loved one. The good news is that sometimes when you change your behavior, your loved one's behaviors will change also. I think you'll be surprised by how much responding with these five steps can improve the outcome of any individual interaction. And over time they just might have a lasting impact.

*H*ow to React in the Middle of a Crisis

No matter how often you get those middle-of-the-night SOS calls, no matter how many times you've found yourself under attack in the middle of what seemed like a civil conversation, every time it happens you're likely to be thrown off balance. Extremely dysregulated behavior has a way of blindsiding you. Frustration and resentment well, or your temper flares, when suddenly confronted by accusations, demands, or agonized pleas. Very few of us react with aplomb in these situations. It's in these circumstances that we most need a quick, automatic response that will dampen, not feed, the flames of emotion. You can practice the five-step response described below until it's a reflex that kicks in the minute you pick up that phone at 4:00 in the morning. But you can also use these steps before or after a crisis, such as when you want to talk to your loved one about a behavior pattern that is hurting her. How to use the five steps in noncrisis situations is discussed on page 91.

Before you get into the five steps, I want you to note that the first step is always to regulate your own emotions. You cannot respond effectively if you are really emotionally upset. Your responses will not be as measured, you will inadvertently say things you wish you hadn't said, and you won't be able to think about what you want to do if you are emotionally dysregulated yourself. So the first thing you should always do in responding to your loved one is to regulate your own emotions. You're probably thinking that's easy for me to say. But there are ways to regulate your own emotion even when you've been caught off guard, detailed below.

The five steps to responding effectively to your loved one appear on the next page. You might want to photocopy the page and keep it where you can review it often until it's committed to memory and as a reminder that this is the best way to communicate in almost all interactions with a person who has borderline personality disorder. Directly following the boxed steps you'll find details on how to carry out each step.

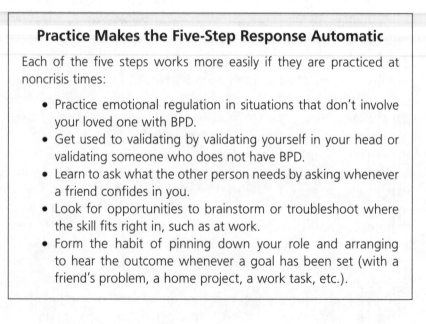

FIVE STEPS TO RESPONDING EFFECTIVELY TO BORDERLINE BEHAVIOR

1. Regulate your own emotion.

2. Validate (do this at every step).

3. Ask/assess.

4. Brainstorm/troubleshoot.

5. Get information on your role (if any) and what you can plan on hearing about the outcome.

Practice Makes the Five-Step Response Automatic

Each of the five steps works more easily if they are practiced at noncrisis times:

- Practice emotional regulation in situations that don't involve your loved one with BPD.
- Get used to validating by validating yourself in your head or validating someone who does not have BPD.
- Learn to ask what the other person needs by asking whenever a friend confides in you.
- Look for opportunities to brainstorm or troubleshoot where the skill fits right in, such as at work.
- Form the habit of pinning down your role and arranging to hear the outcome whenever a goal has been set (with a friend's problem, a home project, a work task, etc.).

Step 1: Regulate Your Own Emotion

A few simple methods can help you dampen emotion in the heat of the moment, but it's easier to put them into action in the middle of a crisis if you've practiced them outside of crisis situations, such as when you're dealing with the frustration of a traffic jam or feeling sadness when a painful memory arises. You might want to photocopy the box on page

74 and carry it with you as a reminder until the steps of regulating your own emotion feel like second nature.

➡ Pause: Take a breath and notice your physical sensations. Label them as the emotion you are experiencing.

"Oh, no! Not again—it's 4:00 in the morning! My heart's suddenly pounding, I instantly have a pain in my gut, and thoughts are rushing through my head. The emotion I'm feeling is ANGER."

➡ Pay attention to your body posture: Unclench your hands, relax the muscles on your face. Make sure your other muscles are not tensed.

"When my sister calls me at 4:00 in the morning, I do a little deep breathing before I even answer the phone (I always know it will be her), and then I make a point of stretching my whole body from the bed after I answer it. It helps focus me on my muscles and not my anger."

➡ Half-smile: Send calming messages to your brain.

"I can't believe how well this works. Along with stretching, it instantly makes me feel calmer."

➡ Validate and cheerlead yourself.

"My emotions are understandable given what is going on."

"I love this person, so of course I have these emotions."

"Emotions make me want to do something to help."

"I accept that I have these emotions about this situation and about my loved one."

**HOW TO REGULATE YOUR EMOTIONS
IN THE HEAT OF THE MOMENT**

Pause.

Pay attention to your body posture.

Half-smile.

Validate and cheerlead yourself.

If you can't regulate your emotions in the moment using the four steps listed in the box, try "opposite action," a useful trick for using actions to change emotions, described in the box on page 75.

If you feel like your own emotions are a big problem in your interactions with your loved one, even when you've been practicing the methods for regulating your emotion, you might take the time to explore what kinds of events and incidents tend to prompt high emotion in you.

Identifying Your Emotional Prompting Events

All of us have situations that make us more emotional than others. We also have times when we have emotional reactions to a situation that we would not normally react to. Use this assessment if you want to identify the "triggers" that cause you to have emotional responses to your loved one. Once you know what makes you more vulnerable to emotions and the situations that spark emotions, you can make decisions about how to change your emotion or when you may choose not to interact with your loved one.

1. Recall a few times when interactions with your loved one went particularly poorly.

2. Did the interactions start off emotionally, did emotions build gradually, or was there an explosion?

3. Were there other things going on in your life that made you more emotional that day? Were you tired, sick, having problems at work? These factors put you at risk for being emotional your-

Linehan's Skill of Opposite Action: Regulating Emotion with Behavior

All emotions have an action—the thing that they propel you to do. If you want to bring that emotion down a little in the moment, use a little opposite action. The four emotions that people experience the most when dealing with interpersonal conflict are fear, anger, guilt, and sadness. I'll discuss fear and guilt in Chapter 11. Here's how you can use the opposite-action technique to regulate anger or sadness.

Anger

Anger makes you want to attack (on the phone, e-mail, in person, text, etc). What's most important to reduce anger is to DISENGAGE. Walk away, hang up, don't text, don't e-mail—but do so gently, without the last word, without ire. Just get distance. If you stay connected, anger will stay up or even increase. After disengaging, practice kindness. See the world through your loved one's eyes, find compassion (see page 96) for him or her, do something kind for him or her. *Anger cannot be maintained in the face of compassion.*

With anger, rumination is often a problem. Cues of anger keep recurring, so compassion has to be used over and over again to keep anger down.

Sadness

Sadness makes you want to isolate yourself and kind of give up, get in bed and pull the covers over your head. It creates inaction. A lot of times, family members of people with BPD wear themselves out trying to help their loved ones, and many times the loved one just remains sad and hopeless. At some point the loved ones get to that place, too. At that point, opposite action is an activation treatment (as opposed to bringing down emotion, it is about bringing up the physiology of the body). Get moving again. If you're trying to lower sadness in the moment, go take a brisk walk. Play tennis. Go for a swim. Put on your aerobic dance DVD. Over the longer term, activate your support system to do pleasant events not related to your loved one (hard, I know, but this will help your loved one), do research into what is available for your loved one, find a support group, and go to one of the family advocacy programs discussed in Chapter 12 and listed at the back of this book. *Do not let your body and your emotions get still and quiet.*

self and will make you less effective in dealing with your loved one.

4. Do a little analysis of the event.

    a. When did it start? This is the prompting event. Most problems have patterns. Look for similar prompting events.

    b. When did it get to the place where the problem between you and your loved one was inevitable? Was there a point of no return?

    c. What happened after the explosion? Did you change your behavior? Did your loved one change his or her behavior? Did you not speak for a few days? What you are looking for is things that might have reinforced your loved one's emotional reaction (like your backing down) or something that might have reinforced your behavior (she got so mad that she didn't talk to you for a few days and you got a break from having to deal with her problems).

For interactions that did not go well, look at the prompting event and your responses. Are there ways that you can change your responses in the moment to deescalate? Did your emotion get in the way? If so, go back to practicing regulating your own emotions. Did you reinforce your loved one's behavior? If so, change your reaction so that it is not reinforcing. You may have to do this several times until you find reactions that are not reinforcing. Were you reinforced for escalating the interaction? If so, think of ways that you can get the desired outcome without escalating.

Step 2: Validate (Do This at Every Step)

➡ **Soothe your loved one's emotions** by finding something to acknowledge (the emotion, the thoughts, the actions).

➡ **Whenever emotion begins to build, stop and validate again.**

For more details and illustrations on how to validate, as well as practice tips, go back to Chapter 3. Here are some quick "rules" to keep in mind:

- Always validate the emotional experience: "I can see that this must hurt a lot." "I can understand why you would be angry about this." (Never say "You shouldn't feel that way," "It can't be that bad," or "Well, look on the bright side ... ")

- Don't correct or contradict your loved one in an attempt to reassure: Say "I know you feel like you're stupid." (Don't go on to say "But you're not.")

- Never validate the invalid: Say "You seem to feel that drinking that much last night wasn't a good idea" instead of "Oh, it's okay; just don't drink that much from now on." Don't say "Well, I guess you just couldn't help it." (This message just confirms your loved one's fears about her incompetence or lack of "self-control" and fragilizes her. Instead, say "What could you do differently to avoid going to the bar next time you feel this way?")

- Whenever in doubt, in fact, ask a question instead of making a statement: "What do you think would work well here?" instead of "You should ... " "Are you feeling disappointed?" instead of "You're obviously disappointed." (People with BPD often object to being told what they are thinking and feeling because they have had such vast experience with being told that the way they feel, think, and act is wrong.)

Step 3: Ask/Assess

▶ **Specifically, but _gently_, ask** "How would you like me to help? Do you want me to listen, give advice, or help you figure out what to do?"

—**If the answer is "Just listen,"** skip STEP 4 (brainstorm/troubleshoot) and move to STEP 5 (get information on your role).

—**If the person wants your input, assess** exactly what is going on:

- What happened?
- When did it start?
- What does your loved one see as the problem?
- What would he/she like to be the outcome after the problem is solved?

Step 4: Brainstorm/Troubleshoot

➧ **Generate a list of solutions** with the help of your loved one.

➧ **Collaborate with your loved one to select an option.**

➧ **Anticipate what could get in the way** of your loved one's actually carrying out the plan.

Step 5: Get Information on Your Role and What You Can Plan on Hearing about the Outcome

➧ **Are there things that you need to do to help/support your loved one** in carrying out the plan?

➧ **Request a check-in/follow-up** if it is important to you. Tell your loved one that you are really interested in knowing what happened and ask to be updated. This is very validating for the person who is in crisis but also doesn't leave you guessing.

What the Five Steps Look Like in Action

Here's a sample script using the five steps. In this scenario, Susan goes to her mom's home, and she is obviously upset.

MOM: What's going on?

SUSAN: You don't really care. You think I deserve everything that happens.

MOM: (*pauses and takes a breath; notices the urge to defend herself but knows that this will not be helpful and will increase Susan's emotions* **[regulating your own emotions]**) Susan, you seem very upset. I'm ready to listen or help if you want. What would you like from me? **[ask]**

SUSAN: (*angry*) I would like for you to make my life better. It sucks.

MOM: I know it does **[validation]**. Tell me what happened.

SUSAN: My boyfriend won't speak to me (*sobbing*).

MOM: That really hurts **[validation]**. I know it does. Do you want to tell me what's going on? **[ask]**

SUSAN: I tried and tried, but he won't call me back.

MOM: Man **[validation]**. Let's talk about this. Do you want me just listening, or do you want me to help you figure out what to try next? **[ask]**

SUSAN: I want your help (*emotion increasing again*).

MOM: (*half-smiles* **[regulating your own emotions]**). Okay, give me the blow-by-blow. Tell me when this started. I'm listening. **[assess]**

SUSAN: Well, we were out last night, and I thought he was looking at another girl. I told him he was a jerk, and he left. Now he won't call me back.

MOM: Okay, do you want me to help you figure out what to do next? **[ask]**

SUSAN: I don't think you can do anything.

MOM: I am not sure I can either. **[validate]** I guess the big question is—and you are the expert on Bruce—do you think it would be more effective to try to get him to talk today or for you to give him some time? **[assess]**

SUSAN: Probably give him time, but I don't think I can handle that.

MOM: What if you and I come up with some things to do while you give him time? **[ask]**

SUSAN: Like what? Go to a movie?

MOM: That's a good start. Let make a list, and then we'll figure out what works best. **[generate solutions]**

Later, after the list is generated:

MOM: Okay, now, do you need me to go with you to the movies **[role clarification]** or do you want to call your friend Callie?

SUSAN: I'll call Callie.

MOM: What if she can't go? What are you going to do then? **[troubleshooting]**

SUSAN: Will you go if she doesn't go?

MOM: Sure, if she does go with you, will you call me after the movie just to let me know how you're doing? **[what you would like to know of the outcome]**

What to Do If Your Loved One Doesn't Participate

Having a five-step plan doesn't guarantee that your loved one will go along with the program, unfortunately. What do you do when he or she doesn't participate? Let's say you've asked how you can help and tried to assess the problem, and she says: "I don't have time to tell you. I need you to fix this now or I'm going to have to kill myself." (*Suicide threats are, sadly, very common among those with BPD. They must be taken seriously, as with anyone else. See Chapter 12 for a discussion of how to respond.*) Or she interrupts you and won't let you ask questions or provide help.

In cases like these, a positive outcome depends greatly on *how well you know yourself* and **how well you know your loved one.** Knowing yourself means first being fully aware of how this turn of events is affecting you. So when your loved one shows no desire to participate, you need to:

➤ **Stop and notice your experience.** Pay attention to your:

➤ Physical sensations

Your stomach (is it tight, clenched, upset, calm?)

Your chest (tight? is breathing slow, shallow, fast?)

Your diaphragm—that place between your ribs (does it feel unsettled?)

Your muscles (are they tight or loose?)

Your hands/fists (clenched or open?)

Your facial muscles (are they wrinkled or smooth?)

Your heart rate (slow or fast?)

➤ Thoughts

"I had a thought that you were not listening to me" as opposed to "You're showing no respect for how I can help you."

➡ Urges   *"I feel like slamming the phone down."*

                                 "I want to scream at you to listen to me."

                                 "I want to rush over to your house to make sure you don't do anything drastic."

➡ Emotions   *"I'm feeling the emotions of anger, frustration, and fear."*

When you pay attention to and label your experience, your emotion immediately begins to regulate. But you also know more about how uncomfortable this situation is making you feel. And that tells you something important that you need to know to respond effectively to a person with BPD: what your limits are and when they are being crossed.

Identifying your limits and knowing when they are being crossed is something that I prefer to call *observing limits*, because I want to stress the need to observe yourself and the circumstances objectively. It's far too easy to view people with BPD as demanding and "manipulative" and therefore deserving of ultimatums, boundary setting, and "drawing the line." When you turn your full awareness to your physical sensations, thoughts, and urges, and then label your emotions, you gather information over time about where you have a true limit. And then you also have enough information to know when that limit is being crossed. You no longer have to subject yourself to seething and stewing until suddenly you've "had it" and impulsively throw up a brick wall against your loved one with BPD.

Observing limits adroitly is a skill developed over time, but it's an important one to cultivate since important personal preferences often seem to get lost in emotionally charged interactions; see page 85 for more details. When your loved one comes to you in crisis but then declines to participate in the five-step approach to keeping emotions in check, you're likely to find yourself needing to consider whether a limit is being crossed and what to do about it. So, once you've stopped to notice your experience, you may need to:

➥ **Communicate a limit to your loved one:**

➥ *Tell him/her that you are going to end the conversation if* _____ *doesn't happen* (you don't lower your voice, you don't let me talk, you keep cursing at me).

➥ *Give him or her a chance, even if it's brief, to modify his or her behavior* to a way of interacting that works for you. This is a very subjective measure. The key is to think about what is reasonable given the case. If your limit is just about this one interaction ("I want you to stop telling me I don't care about you"), you give just a couple of chances ("You're doing it again. I want you to stop"). If your limit is about multiple interactions ("Every time you disagree with me, you walk out and slam the door"), you will give longer. It may take a couple of similar situations before you get your loved one to quit slamming the door. The key is to make sure there is time to change the behavior.

➥ *Make sure you "own" that you are ending the interaction because of your reactions and what you want from the interaction.*

"I know this is painful for you, but it's what I need to be able to stay in our relationship."

"I can't do this right now because I have so much going on at work and I don't have the time to give you."

"I know I used to take calls from you all the time, but now you are calling 20 times a day. I have realized that 20 times is just too many for me."

➥ *YOU ACTUALLY HAVE TO FOLLOW THROUGH.* If you say that you're going to stop the conversation if the behavior doesn't change and it does not, do what you said you were going to do (or you will inadvertently reinforce the behavior you wanted to stop).

➥ *WHY IT'S SO IMPORTANT TO KNOW YOUR LOVED ONE*: If your loved one's refusal to participate includes threats of self-harm, you obviously have to know the person and what is reinforcing for him or her to know how to respond. You would never cavalierly say "I'm not going to talk to you anymore" and hang up on someone who has just said she is going to kill herself. But if you know from experience that allowing your limit to be crossed without consequence encourages the other person to keep doing what you find intolerable, you have to find a different response. To the woman who says, "I need you to fix this right now or I'm going to kill myself," you might say "Okay, then I'm calling the police." If she is seriously contemplating suicide, then calling the police is the right thing to do anyway. But a good portion of the time, those with BPD will say that killing themselves is not in fact what they want. This allows you to go back to **asking and assessing**, all while restating your limit and at the same time **validating** how your having communicated this limit feels to her:

➡ **Validate and soothe your loved one's emotions about having the limit established.**

➡ **Assure your loved one that you will be available at a different time or for different issues.**

What Responding to Nonparticipation Looks Like in Action

I had a client once who would call and scream at me on the telephone. When I tried to speak, she would talk over me and curse at me. Then she would hang up and I would be worried that she was going to kill herself. Finally I noticed that I was feeling dread whenever the phone rang and that when I was on the phone with her I had the urge to hang up the phone. I labeled the emotion as frustration and noticed that it really hurt my feelings.

First I had a conversation with the client where I described what was happening: "Each time that you have called me recently you have yelled at me, cursed at me, and hung up on me. Now I am noticing that when my telephone rings, I experience dread that it will be a call from you. I don't think that you are calling with the goal of hanging up on me and know that you are really,

really upset when you call, but it hurts my feelings and makes me feel like an inadequate therapist. If we can't get these calls to go in such a way that I feel better, I am going to have to quit taking calls from you."

At this point, she became dysregulated and told me that I was only thinking of myself. I validated this, told the truth (it was about me), and kept moving. "I know this is not what you want to hear. Here's another person not wanting to talk with you. It's like the pattern of your life. But you're right: this is about me. I don't like to be interrupted, cursed at, or hung up on when I am on the phone. I like to be listened to and appreciated. That's just how I am. The thing is, we've got to work this out or I will quit taking calls after hours."

After I got her to listen, I told her exactly what I wanted. I wanted her to let me talk, not curse, and not hang up on me. I gave her a few weeks to at least make progress. I told her repeatedly that I knew this was hard on her and reminded her that this was about what I wanted on the telephone. Ultimately, she did not stop. At that point I told her that she could not call me after 5:00 P.M. until calls earlier in the day demonstrated that she had changed her behavior (giving her a different way to have access to me). It took her several months, but her behavior changed. As soon as it did, I allowed her to call again at night, and my limits were no longer crossed.

What to Do If Your Loved One Attacks or Gets Extremely Emotional

Remember, a major goal of the five-step response is to regulate emotion. If your loved one declines to participate and doesn't hear your validation or take the time to answer your questions, his emotions are likely to keep spiraling out of control. Sometimes you might find that despite your attempts to respond helpfully you end up attacked. In these cases:

➡ **1. Stop and regulate your emotions (see page 72).**

Hold ice in your hands if you can get to it (it will dampen your urges to attack back).

➡ 2. For a few minutes, do nothing but validate:

Restate what your loved one is saying.	*"So, you were at work and your boss wanted to talk with you. You were really, really anxious."*
Say things that sound interested and caring.	*"I understand; tell me more."*
Ask questions.	*"What happened next?"*
Normalize SOMETHING in his/her response.	*"It's really upsetting just talking about it. It's tough. I know this is hard. It would be hard for anyone."*

➡ 3. Go back to what you were doing (problem solving, giving advice, etc.) before the outburst.

➡ The key here is to stop and validate until the emotion subsides. Enough validation and anyone is going to run out of steam with the emotion. It may go up again in a moment, but then you stop and validate again.

> *If you feel like finding something in your loved one's behavior to normalize will require you to make something up, it might help to remember that there is what we do naturally and then there's what we need to do strategically.*

*I*dentifying and Communicating Limits

All of us have personal limits, and it's our job to maintain them. The crises in the lives of people with BPD and the lengths that we will go to to help the people we love often result in our limits being stretched and crossed, as discussed earlier in this chapter. Unfortunately, research is really clear that there is a point of no return with limits. When they are pushed too far, they and the relationship are irreparable. So that that doesn't happen, we have to know where our limits are. The tough thing is that we don't know where our limits are until someone/something pushes up against them. For this reason, we need to observe to know our limits. The steps for regulating your own emotion (see page 72) show you how to observe your internal processes. Pay attention to your physical sensations, your thoughts, your action urges. Have you ever noticed that your body clenched whenever you were around a particular person or that you experienced dread at the thought of being with that person or that when the phone rang you didn't want to pick it up? You were observing. If you knew what caused that reaction (she called too late, too often, cursed too much in front of you, berated or criticized, said hurtful things), you would observe that you have a limit (you don't like to be called after 10:00 P.M., called more than four times a day, cursed at, berated or criticized, have hurtful things said about you). You would have to decide whether the relationship was important enough to you and whether you wanted to "communicate those limits" to the person.

Practicing Spotting Your Limits

We all have lots of limits that we don't articulate clearly. Before you start actively observing yourself to identify limits, it might help to try identifying some of your unarticulated limits, including ones that have nothing to do with the person with BPD that you love. Ask yourself:

- Do you have limits about your loved one coming to your home?
    If so, when is it all right for your loved one to visit?
    When is it not all right for your loved one to visit?
- Do you have limits about phone calls with friends?
    With family?
    With your loved one with BPD?
- What are your physical limits with touch with your loved one?
- What are your limits with language and emotionality (are you a person who can tolerate cursing, loud speaking, physical agitation)?

Using "Pros and Cons" to Make Decisions about Communicating That a Limit Has Been Crossed

In DBT, we use a four-way pros-and-cons analysis to help people make decisions in a wise fashion. At first glance, it would seem that these would repeat themselves, but they generate very different solutions. I'm going to do a pros and cons about whether to take telephone calls on Friday nights from my sister after she has been out drinking and calls my home after midnight.

	Taking the Calls	Not Taking the Calls
Pros	She's not angry on Sat. Phone doesn't ring all night Know she's at home	Don't get yelled at Can spend time with husband Won't be mad at her
Cons	Ruins my night My husband gets upset I feel out of control	I will worry about her She'll call my mom She'll leave 100 voice mails

There is no right or wrong interpretation of the pros and cons, and it is not about adding up the different quadrants. It is about finding the "wise" answer for yourself. As I look at these pros and cons, to me it leans toward the cons of taking the calls and the pros of not taking the calls. If possible, I would have a conversation with my sister in advance and explain what my limits are and that I will not answer the phone when she calls after a certain time on Friday nights.

The process of identifying and communicating limits is summed up below. Consider photocopying it and carrying it with you as you begin the process of observing limits effectively.

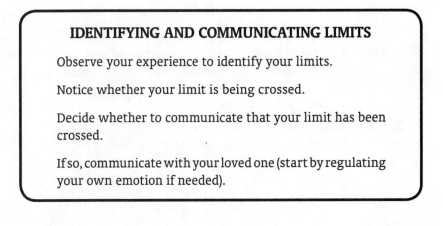

IDENTIFYING AND COMMUNICATING LIMITS

Observe your experience to identify your limits.

Notice whether your limit is being crossed.

Decide whether to communicate that your limit has been crossed.

If so, communicate with your loved one (start by regulating your own emotion if needed).

How to Communicate a Limit ahead of Time

As in the example of my sister's Friday night phone calls, most of the time you'll do best if you communicate ahead of time about a limit you've identified:

➡ **1. Make sure you know your own limits.**

➡ **2. Don't talk with your loved one about your limits when she is already emotionally distressed about something. At this point, she is vulnerable and the response is bound to be negative. Describe the facts of the situation—usually it helps to have a recent event that everyone will remember.**

"On Friday nights when you go to happy hour, you often call me when you get home. Last Friday night, you called me four times after 10:00."

➡ **3. Express your feelings about this situation while also validating and soothing your loved one.**

"I enjoy talking with you, but I really want to have Friday nights with my husband. It really frustrates me when you call and you've had too much to drink."

➡ **4. State the limit.**

"So, I don't want you to call me after the bars on Friday night anymore."

➡ **5. Anticipate an emotional increase and move in to soothe and validate.**

"I know you are lonely when you come home to the big old apartment on Friday nights and it's hard not to have someone to talk to."

➧ **6. You can now move into using the five steps to act and react outside of a crisis and problem-solve what your loved one can do to avoid crossing your limit while doing something helpful for herself.**

"What do you think you could do on a Friday night when you're lonely?"

Tips for Communicating Limits Effectively

• No matter what happens next, keep repeating some version of your limit ("I don't want you to call me after going to the bar"), along with some validation.

• Remember that limits are about you, not about your loved one. *Communicate this.* Recognize that life might be better for your sister if she could call at 10:00 P.M. after she got home from the bars. It certainly wouldn't get worse. Don't act as if limits are for her good. Limits are not. They are for your good.

• Make sure you soothe your loved one when you communicate a limit. Limits are hard and kind of devastating. If possible, offer something else. In the case of the Friday night telephone calls, you could say "I know you really want to talk with me on Friday night and I really want to hear what is going on with you. Why don't you call me on Saturday morning when you wake up and we will debrief Friday night."

• Validate how hard it is to have someone withdraw something. Say, "I know it's hard for you because you really want to talk with me on Friday night and it's hard to hear someone say you can't do what you want." Or "It's hard to have someone tell you you can't call when you want to."

• Be honest about what you are doing and why. Don't tell your sister that the reason she can't call is that your husband is making you do it.

How to Stick to Your Guns When Communicating Limits

• Remind yourself that giving in if your loved one gets upset when you communicate a limit will reinforce your loved one's escalated emotions. (Similarly, if you take the inevitable calls next Friday night, you are reinforcing that behavior.)

• Keep in mind that it's likely to be painful for your loved one to hear about your limit, and your loved one's pain is likely to bring up emotions in you that will make you want to reconsider. Let's say you've paid your brother's rent for several months and now realize you don't have the money to do so anymore. You have "observed" that you have a limit and you need to communicate it to your brother. When you tell your brother that you cannot pay the rent any longer, he will undoubtedly react emotionally. It could be that the emotion is anger that you won't pay anymore or fear that there will be no way for him to pay the rent. Those emotions may begin to persuade you to give in and pay the rent. Now you'll want to revisit your limits. It could be that there is some money to pay the rent for a few extra months. Or maybe you're willing to take some phone calls in the middle of the night. Usually, the problem is that your loved one's emotions (and resulting actions—tears, threats) are influencing your emotions.

The typical emotions that people feel when communicating limits are guilt ("I shouldn't have said that. She needs this more than I do. I hurt her"), shame ("I should be a better parent/husband/friend"), and fear ("If I don't do this, she may kill herself"). These emotional responses are discussed further in Chapter 11. For now, know that if you back down on your limits out of your own emotion, you will reinforce your loved one's emotional reaction. More important, you'll be edging close to burning out on the relationship. If you con-

> Limits are hard to communicate, but they keep you in the relationship.

tinue to change your limits, resentment will grow in you. Think about a situation where you really did not like what someone was doing. Think about what you really wanted to tell that person or a limit that you wanted to communicate but didn't. What ultimately happened? Most often, there is an explosion at some point where you just hit your limit with the behavior. Many times, that ultimate explosion results in the relationship ending.

• Use the "broken record" technique when communicating a limit. This means repeating yourself verbatim. It gives you something to be mindful of—the repetition of your limits, the soothing statements, and so on—and it keeps your emotion tamped down. Remind yourself of the benefits of communicating the limits. If you have done a pros-and-cons analysis, repeat to yourself the results of the pros and cons. The important thing is to repeatedly tell yourself the end result if you don't communicate the limit.

• Know the difference between giving in on a limit and changing it because the circumstances have changed. When you think of a limit as being a boundary, you'll find that it feels set in stone. Historically, therapists and talk-show hosts have talked about the need to "set boundaries" with people with BPD. But today we don't use the word *boundaries*. Boundaries are walls. They are impermeable and inflexible. Once you set a boundary, it cannot be changed. We use *limits* because we see them as flexible and able to change with circumstances. Limits change with time, between people, and with situations. My limits with my husband are different from those with my mother, which are different from those with my coworkers. My limits around being accessible to clients with BPD are usually pretty open, but if my partner were having back surgery and needed me to care for him for a few weeks, my limits would be temporarily different. I wouldn't be as available as I usually am.

Limits can change due to circumstances. If something catastrophic is happening in your loved one's life (she works for a company that is going out of business and laying people off), you may extend limits that you usually have. For instance, if you have a "don't drop by the house without calling first" limit, you may, for that period of time when the layoffs are occurring and until your loved one gets a new job, relax that limit. Of course, if your loved one begins to drop by every day and at inopportune moments, you may have to communicate some limits, even around the temporarily extended limits. The key is to see limits as fluid and changeable.

*H*ow to Act and React Outside of a Crisis

People with BPD tend to get trapped in patterns of destructive or self-destructive behavior. When you care about one of them, it's awfully hard to watch the same mistakes being made over and over. Yet it's also hard to find a way to talk about these problems without triggering emotional upheaval in your loved one. Maybe you hate seeing your brother engage in risky sexual behavior and want to talk to him at a calm moment about how he could make more self-protective choices. Or maybe your daughter comes to you matter of factly and wants to talk about what's been going on with her boyfriend. With or without BPD in the mix, you would hope that you could have a constructive discussion about these issues in your loved one's life. Your fondest wish might be that gradually your loved one could begin to chip away at a problem that's been interfering with his or her happiness or even safety.

Unfortunately, even in the absence of BPD, such discussions can push too many buttons and end without improving the situation—or possibly even make things worse. But *with* BPD in the mix, your brother might get extremely emotional if he feels criticized. Or as you talk to your daughter, thinking you're having a good conversation, something could set her off and you could find yourself suddenly accused of causing all the trouble because you never liked the guy. Because of the potential emotional charge, it's especially important to use the five steps to respond in a way that will keep emotions under control and pave the way for problems to be solved.

The steps are the same as when you use them in the middle of a crisis. But when a crisis isn't imminent, you reach a fork in the road at Step 3:

➡ **3. Ask:** "Can I help you?" or "Do you want my help?"

"Yes"	"No"
↓	↓

Assess:

What is going on? Get an accurate picture of where the issue started, when it started, and who is needed to solve the problem.

Validate your loved one's point of view.

Accept being unable to help.

Approach your loved one about the problem again later.

Identify and communicate a limit if the continuation of this behavior makes it necessary.

If Your Loved One Wants Your Help ...

Your task is to proceed with Steps 4 and 5, doing your best to communicate in a way that is supportive and encouraging without being over the top: Give low-key (not over-the-top, fragilizing) encouragement that your loved one can do what you have planned. Think of yourself as a coach. Your loved one is still the athlete and could compete without you, but things will go much better if you are on the sidelines.

When you ask in Step 4 what role you should play, be explicit:

"Should I help directly?"
"Do you want me to be a cheerleader on the sideline?"
"Do you want me just to wait to hear how things turn out?"

In Step 5, express interest in the outcome:

"I would really like to hear how this turns out."
"Will you check in with me and let me know how it goes?"

Throughout the five-step process, if your loved one's emotions increase, back down a little and validate a lot. When the emotions subside, move back in with problem solving. If *your* emotions increase, go back to the tips for bringing your own emotions down (page 72).

If Your Loved One Does Not Want Your Help ...

You might have to work on cultivating acceptance. Compassion and acceptance, discussed in the following section, are enormously helpful when dealing with someone with BPD.

If you find yourself feeling very sad about having your offer of help declined, try the "opposite-action" technique described in the box on page 75.

It could be that you go through all of the steps in regulating yourself and offering help to your loved one and she not only refuses your help but becomes more dysregulated. At that point, acceptance and self-compassion are the way to keep yourself from falling into the emotional and behavioral abyss with your loved one.

*P*racticing Acceptance and Self-Compassion

We are often told that we cannot change other people. As a behaviorist, I believe that we have some capacity to change others by changing our reactions to others. Most of this book talks about how to do that. At the end of the day, however, a lot of acceptance is needed in dealing with our loved ones.

In DBT, we teach that misery is caused by pain (emotional or physical) plus nonacceptance of that pain. Pain is a part of life and definitely a part of dealing with other people. We cannot have relationships that are pain free. However, it is when we do not accept the current reality that we escalate from pain to misery.

Think of putting your hand on a hot stove burner. The stove burns your hand. Nonacceptance is not moving your hand and leaving it on the burner. You are crying out, "My hand hurts. It's burning." Nothing changes until you accept that your hand is on the stove. Then you move your hand. Often, we just keep talking about how badly our hand hurts and we never accept that our hand is on the stove and the stove is on.

In every moment, we need to accept reality as it is. We need to accept

1. Our loved one as he or she is in this moment.
2. Our reactions to our loved one as he or she is in this moment.
3. The situation at hand.

To be clear, accepting these things doesn't mean that we don't wish it were different and that we won't work really hard to change the next moment. What it means is that we are clearly seeing reality as it is.

People often think that they have to accept the future. They say, "I have to accept that she will never change." YOU DO NOT HAVE TO ACCEPT THE FUTURE. You only have to accept this moment. I worked one time with women who were incarcerated and had BPD. Most of them had committed tragic crimes and had life sentences. They would ask me how they could accept that they would be in prison until they died. The answer was that they did not have to accept being in prison until they died. They had to accept being in prison right then. That day. The next day, of course, they would have to accept being in prison again. And the next day. And the next day. Acceptance for them had to repeated over and over.

You have to accept your loved one right where she is right now. Tomorrow you may have to accept that she is the same way. Or she may be different tomorrow and you will have to accept her then. Equally important, you have to accept yourself right where you are now. Tomorrow you may have to accept that you are the same way. Or you may be different tomorrow and you will have to accept yourself then.

Acceptance of yourself means accepting your emotions. You are bound to have many emotions about your loved one. Sadness that her life did not turn out as you would have wished. Fear that he will do something catastrophic. Anger that she is hurting herself and you. Disappointment in his situation. Guilt that you did not do certain things at certain times to help your loved one. Whatever your emotions are, when they arise, it is important that you accept them. You have to acknowledge their existence. Only after you acknowledge them can you either continue to accept the emotions or work to change them.

A note on the word *practice* that is used with acceptance. There are some things that we just accept. If you wake up one morning and you don't want to go to work that day, you may accept that it's Wednesday and that you have to go to work. Then you get up and go to work. However, the acceptance that we are talking about here is more problematic than acceptance of Wednesday and work. The acceptance here is of painful things. We use the word *practice* as an acknowledgment that there is no magical place called "acceptance" that you arrive at where things are not as painful. Instead, we keep working and working at acceptance, so we use the word *practicing* acceptance instead of *getting to* acceptance in acknowledgment of the journey.

How Do You Practice Acceptance?

You can practice acceptance in the heat of the moment with your loved one when you notice that you are holding on to an idea or an emotion and it is causing you discomfort, or you can practice it when you are not interacting with your loved one. Many times, you will have pain from previous interactions or distress about current life situations that will require practicing acceptance.

1. Determine what you are not accepting. Ask yourself, what is making me miserable?
2. State out loud: "I accept. ... "
3. Pay attention to your body posture. Make sure you have an accepting posture:
   a. Make sure your hands are not clenched.
   b. Relax your facial muscles.

Compassion as Acceptance

One of the sure ways to keep your emotions in check is to practice compassion, which, of course, requires acceptance of yourself and your loved one. There are formal Buddhist practices called *loving-kindness meditations* that are really helpful in developing compassion for others. However, you can practice the acceptance and emotional regulation by developing compassion. Compassion allows you to experience empathy with others' difficulties. It's important not to confuse compassion and empathy with pity. Pity will make you treat your loved one as if she is hopeless or fragile and will not be helpful. Pity often has some judgment in it as opposed to acceptance ("I feel so sorry for her because …"). Compassion is deep-rooted acceptance of the person as he or she is in the moment.

Compassion starts with self-compassion. You cannot accept another person and have compassion for him if you don't have compassion for yourself. It's hard to have compassion in the heat of the moment, so you have to practice it before emotions are high.

Ways to Practice Compassion

1. Start with yourself:

    a. Visualize yourself as joyous and accepting. What does that look like? See a half-smile on your face. Visualize yourself doing kind things. Picture yourself responding to situations with patience and skill.

    b. Think of your positive qualities. What are some of your past acts of kindness? When were you accepting of someone even in the face of unpleasantness?

    c. Make statements out loud that are compassionate, accepting statements of yourself. These can be affirmations but also can be statements of fact about past compassionate moments ("I have put myself in her shoes and realized how difficult it is for her to feel like she is losing everything even when she was yelling at me that she hated me"). Find things about yourself to love and say them over and over again.

2. Now, try the same thing with your loved one. It may be helpful to write down what works in the different ways of practicing compassion.

a. Visualize: picture your loved one being joyous and unburdened. What does this look like?

_____

_____

b. Think of positive qualities of your loved one and kind, compassionate things that he has done in his life:

_____

_____

_____

c. Make statements out loud that are compassionate, accepting statements of your loved one. Choose the statements that bring you acceptance (a feeling of peace) and turn these into statements that you can commit to memory.

_____

_____

_____

Self-Care as Self-Compassion

One way to take care of your relationship with your loved one is to care for yourself. In addition to developing an accepting, compassionate stance about yourself, you need to take care of your body and your emotions. Having a healthy body will make you stronger and less vulnerable to experiencing emotions even when your loved one is emotional. There are several ways to do this:

• First, *take care of your physical self.* Make sure you eat well, sleep well, avoid too much caffeine, alcohol, and sugar. Take time off from work to recharge yourself. Find things to do that bring you pleasure and make you feel in control. These things will decrease your emotional reactivity.

• *Soothe your senses.* Experts have found that people who self-soothe every day are less irritable than people who don't self-soothe. Making sure that you soothe your senses is one way to keep your emotions down. Take some time every day to do little things that take the edge off your emotions. Think of the five senses:

Touch: take a warm bath, snuggle with your pets, touch soft blankets

Taste: eat soothing foods, put soothing tastes in your mouth (caramel), drink warm tea, cocoa, coffee

Smell: create a relaxing, spalike scent in your home or space with lavender, eucalyptus, flowers, cinnamon, candles

Sight: look at things that bring you calm. The water, the mountains, pictures, children playing

Sound: listen to soothing music, surf sounds, cats purring

• *Take a little vacation.* Vacations are all about healing and fortifying ourselves so that we are refueled for life. Take a few hours for yourself. Sit outside in a lawn chair, watch sports, read a novel. Do something that you can do without worrying or ruminating about the past or the future. Just take a break. You will be less vulnerable to emotions at the end of the break.

One way to get through difficult situations is to cheerlead yourself. Many of us are really good at telling others that they can get through situations or building them up when under duress but not good at doing so for ourselves. If you are one of those people:

1. Think of what you would say if a friend called and told you of a situation that was similar to yours.
2. List three things that you would say to cheerlead your friend.
3. Repeat those three things to yourself each day until they become statements that you can say automatically.

Now that you have step-by-step methods for responding to the out-of-control behaviors and emotions of your loved one, we will begin to look at exactly what some of those behaviors are. In the next section, we will examine six specific behavioral patterns in people with BPD and give illustrations for how to use regulation and acceptance with each.

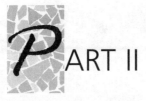

PART II

The Many Faces of Borderline Personality Disorder

"I Can't Stand Feeling Like This!"

"I'm about to lose Jack! I'm *sure* of it. I can't stand how much this hurts. I won't make it if I lose him."

This is what Dana's older sister heard one night when she answered her phone at 11:00, and then at 1:00, and finally at 4:00 A.M.. Dana was certain that she was losing her husband because she had yelled at him several times during the day, accused him of having affairs, cried, and threatened to kill herself. Gail had tried to reassure Dana that Jack loved her and wouldn't leave her. She'd tried distracting her with other topics. She had given her whatever advice seemed likely to calm her sister down. But Dana was spiraling into a vortex that kept pulling her deeper and deeper into despair. With no idea how to get out, she kept demanding that Gail pull her free.

Gail was tired. Not just due to lack of sleep on that night but because they'd been through all this before. Periodically, with very little warning, something would seem to set Dana off and she'd get caught up in a mode where she was ruled by intense emotions and certain she was doomed to be this way for the rest of her life. She'd feel—and act—totally out of control and helpless. At one moment she'd plead for her sister's help. Then she'd lash out at Gail, accusing her of not caring at all no matter what kind of support Gail tried to give. Then she'd descend to the depths and say her only choice was to end it all—nothing would ever change and she just couldn't stand it anymore.

If you love someone with BPD, this manifestation of the disorder may be very familiar to you since emotional dysregulation is such a core aspect of BPD. And, of course, we've discussed emotional dysregulation as if it's a constant in those with BPD. In actuality it's not a constant *state*. What is constant for those with BPD is *emotional vulnerability*. At any time your loved one is vulnerable to becoming emotionally dysregulated. Most people with BPD go through periods of relative emotional calm. Often, however, they get sucked into an emotional vortex and may stay there for days or even weeks. It's this behavior that I want to talk about in this chapter. You may find it easier to deal with this primary BPD behavior if you understand why the cycle occurs.

You know from Chapter 2 that people with BPD are naturally emotional and have learned to distrust and discount their emotions. This double whammy leaves them vulnerable not only to experiencing extreme emotions but also to having an extreme *reaction* to feeling emotionally out of control. This is how the whirlpool starts swirling.

In Dana's case, Gail doesn't know what started her sister's journey into the abyss. In fact Dana doesn't understand it either. But once she gets into that dark hole, her emotions just seem to build and build, and then Dana gets more and more upset not by whatever set off her emotions in the first place *but by feeling like she has no ability to stop them.*

I think of this phenomenon as a whirlpool or quicksand because it's something that snares your loved one periodically—possibly quite often—but is not his or her constant state. It couldn't be. Relentless emotional pain at that level really would be difficult to survive (which is why suicide is, tragically, not uncommon among those with BPD; see Chapter 12). Most people with BPD pull themselves from the whirlpool and return to a tolerable emotional state, sometimes with effective behaviors, sometimes with dysfunctional behaviors, and most often by moving into self-invalidation, which is discussed in Chapter 6. I have met people with BPD who have lives that seem to be nothing but despair yet still have moments when they believe there may be ways to extricate themselves.

Because people with BPD often *don't* know what has set off their emotions once the whirlpool starts spinning, you may have very little idea where danger lies for your loved one, either in the world at large or in your one-on-one interactions. And it may not really matter to you. Figuring out the complex chain of emotions and behaviors that entraps those with BPD is a job for qualified professionals. You may have exhausted yourself tiptoeing around in a futile effort to shut down *all* potential emotional stimuli, and still the vortex opens up and grabs your loved one more often than either of you can stand. The good news is that you can dampen the emotional fires that flare up in your loved one by modifying your *own* reactions. As you'll see, you may very well learn something about the themes and patterns involved in triggering your loved one's emotions in the process.

The Anatomy of an Emotional Whirlpool

Let's take a closer look at this whirlpool and how it draws your loved one—and then you—in.

Your Loved One's Experience

Usually, something happens that is painful to the person with BPD. For the moment, whether it would be painful for you or someone who does not have BPD doesn't matter. What is important is that the event causes the person with BPD to have a strong emotional reaction. The pain goes on and on. It seems uncontrollable, unstoppable. This experience of pain becomes overwhelming. This is when the person with BPD is in despair. As this continues, hopelessness blossoms. For the person you love, there seems to be nowhere to go with these emotions. She's standing on a precipice, and all she can see is an eternity of pain and despair. When hopeless, your partner or parent or child or brother sees no way out of the current situation and sees a future of nothing but pain.

Marie is 45 years old and has met the diagnostic criteria for BPD. She and her partner have a child together. Marie says she has been hurt over and over by her partner and her child, who is 5. Her partner says she is not trying to hurt Marie and, in fact, she is trying hard *not* to say anything that has any chance of hurting her. Marie thinks of herself as on emotional overload and experiences everything as one more instance of people hurting her. Marie's pain is excruciating and seems unending to her to the point that she will do anything to shut it down. No matter what anyone says to her to try to lessen her pain (whether it is trying to help her solve the problems that are causing her pain or just trying to communicate understanding of her pain), it is hurtful to her and she begins to tell her partner that she cannot take

> Hopelessness is the enemy of those with BPD and of those who love them.

any more of the pain that she is dishing out to her. She is experiencing pain plus the pain of being in pain simultaneously. Marie sees no way out of the pain and believes that she will feel this way forever.

The whirlpool of emotional vulnerability often starts with some event that your loved one finds hurtful, frightening, confusing, or distressing in some other way. As I said, to understand this particular mechanism you don't really need to know exactly what that event was (to solve their problems, however, those with BPD do eventually need to come to some understanding of the prompting event). What you do need to understand is that an emotion that would subside and be reconciled in the mind of a person without BPD is perpetuated in your loved one. The whirlpool pulls in other emotions and behaviors, becoming a long stream of behavior that ends up with the person with BPD engaging in some impulsive behavior in a desperate attempt to kill the pain. Marie turns to alcohol on some occasions; she also binges and purges. Then her own behavior causes her to react with another uncomfortable emotion, often shame and guilt: First she can't control her emotions, and now she can't control her actions. In her own mind she is beneath contempt.

Another common secondary emotion is anger. Let's say your cousin who has BPD is supposed to come to dinner at your house. Instead, he has been sitting at home alone all day and cannot find the energy to get dressed and come over. You call him and ask where he is. He feels shame and guilt about not being at your house, and he was already feeling very sad and lonely. Now the emotion of anger comes up in a very strong way. This anger acts as an escape valve that shuts down the shame, guilt, sadness, and loneliness because it is powerful and full of energy. Anger allows your cousin to avoid those other emotions, which he finds much less acceptable—and therefore much more painful—than anger. But then he snaps at you out of anger, and that behavior makes him again feel ashamed and guilty. His emotions escalate; the whirlpool spins ever faster, and its downward pull gets ever stronger. He feels more and more out of control, which makes him more and more emotional.

You can see how complicated and self-perpetuating this cycle can become. This complexity is one reason your loved one can stay caught in the emotional whirlpool for days or even weeks. Typically the impulsive behavior that's an attempt to avoid painful emotion causes its own emotional reaction and lands many people in an ongoing state of crisis. When the crisis—a feud with a family member, a bender or a binge, a spending spree or scrapes with the law—remains unresolved, it, too, fuels the whirlpool.

It's not, however, just events and emotions that can get the whirlpool started and keep it going. It's also memories. People with BPD have an active memory of pain. They tend to focus on anniversaries and memories of painful events, thanks to the very plastic brain that we all have. We all learn through experience. Let's say you go to a carnival and have a great time; your brain will form a positive association with carnivals. When you encounter something that reminds you of a carnival, you might feel happy and excited. But what if you went to a carnival and were frightened by a clown? Your brain would form a negative association with carnivals and clowns. Seeing a picture of a clown might reignite that fear. Riding past a street carnival might refire that fear. This fear might be perfectly functional if either carnivals or clowns were a real threat to your life. But it would be dysfunctional if you had a panic attack when a clown arrived at your child's birthday party. Just like with that carnival or clown, the brain of a person with BPD forms negative associations with emotions, which are often overly intense and therefore uncomfortable at the very least. The person with BPD has also come to view these emotions as unacceptable, contributing to the negative association. This is how the experience of one negative emotion can fire another, as with the man whose anger is triggered when he feels shame over not coming to your house for dinner.

Emotions love emotions. Negative emotions love negative emotions. People with BPD are like sponges for pain. They absorb anything negative, and they perceive that there is no way to get out of the tragedy of their lives. The emotions build and build, and the ultimate state that results in that building of negative emotion is hopelessness. Hopelessness is the enemy of your loved one and you: Risk of suicide goes up with increased hopelessness and/or anger. It's a way that people with BPD can say "I'll show you how badly I'm hurting."

Your Reaction—and Where It Leads

Typically, people watching someone they love being sucked into an emotional vortex go into one of two modes: "fixing" or "protecting." We all tend to want to jump in and fix things that aren't working for the people we love. That instinct is even stronger when we see the person we love experiencing emotional agony. You've probably made herculean efforts to try to "fix" whatever is hurting your loved one. Why, then, do all your efforts seem to fail—or make things worse?

You've probably seen your attempts to "cheer up" the other person fall flat. Maybe they've made your loved one angry. Ever stood there totally confused as you feel intense anger radiating from your loved one when you've offered numerous reassurances and positive suggestions, all in good faith and love? It's not because you aren't helpful enough or loving enough. Usually, the person with BPD is angry at you for not understanding how much pain he is in and angry at himself for being so emotional and/or for being unable to solve the problem for himself. To someone with BPD, any response that doesn't validate his experience of pain is unsympathetic. So trying to help him solve the problem is validating only if you acknowledged how much pain the problem is causing. Trying to downplay the magnitude of the problem, on the other hand, is invalidating of how much pain the problem is causing your loved one. Trying to reassure him that he can solve the problem is invalidating of the shame or guilt he feels at not having been able to do so thus far. *As you learned in Chapters 3 and 4, validating the person's emotional experience first and foremost is essential.*

Maybe you're familiar with the sequence of events where your loved one becomes more and more despondent, you make suggestions, and she then tells you all the reasons why your advice would not work. If you told her things were going to get better, she became angry and said something to the effect of "You don't know anything!" If you left her alone, she told you that you didn't care about her or how much pain she was in.

You, of course, start worrying that you cannot say anything without causing trouble, so you try to protect your loved one—as Marie's partner did with Marie—by saying nothing. Then your loved one, as Marie did with her partner, tells you that saying nothing is hurtful also. You've hit the "catch-22" of BPD.

When people with BPD are extremely emotional, what they want to know from others is that their level of pain is understandable. Their experience has generally been the opposite: that their emotions are so over the top that they are *not* understandable. They are frightened by their own emotions (of course, so are we) and simultaneously so exquisitely sensitive to any communication that they are overreacting. They are feeling totally out of control and very sensitive to any communication that they need to be in control. They have no hope for themselves and are afraid you have no hope for them either. They're drowning in their own emotions and watching themselves flounder.

If they've had some DBT, they may be acutely aware that they have a history of being invalidated. They get that they're causing a problem, that they're a freight train out of control, but that doesn't mean they know how to stop it any more than a freight train with no brakes can stop itself.

As to protective mode, it just doesn't work, and it exhausts you in the process. Thirty-year-old Stacy was living with her parents when she found herself about to lose her job as an emergency services dispatcher because she had "lost" it with her supervisor on a number of occasions. She had tremendous emotional responses to the stories that she heard while dispatching, and she would often allow emotions from one call affect her ability to concentrate on subsequent calls. After being written up at work and given a warning that she would be terminated, she retreated to her room and didn't come out for days. Her parents didn't know how to respond. They tried leaving her alone, but she seemed to be even more despondent. She was upset with them because they weren't talking with her about her job. Finally, her parents tried to "have a talk" with her. Stacy's parents tried to be very, very gentle with her. Her reaction escalated, and Stacy accused her parents of treating her like a child.

Once you realize that all your attempts to fix your loved one's problems don't dampen the emotions and might even make them worse, you might naturally decide to just try to create a stress-free, calm, nonantagonistic environment for your loved one. This might mean your taking on all the difficult tasks that any family has to deal with—caring for the ill, handling financial problems, resolving interpersonal conflicts, preparing for an uncertain future. Doing this depletes the physical, financial, and emotional resources of even the strongest among us.

But remember, it's not just the events that occur in your loved one's life that can trigger emotions and kick the maelstrom into action. You can't protect your loved one from her own experiences of pain. And if you don't know how certain events make your loved one feel, you may put a lot of effort into protecting her from things that don't bother her and inadvertently expose her to events that are exceedingly disturbing to her after all. Remember that high emotionality affects the way we process information. So, your loved one may be prone to misinterpreting facts. There's not much you can do to change that propensity by trying to orchestrate her life to excise influences that would cause *you* or others without BPD emotional pain. It's like leaving the lights on for a child who's afraid of the dark: You still have no control over how a shadow cast by a piece of furniture is going to look to a frightened little kid, and the child never learns that the dark is not threatening.

> *You may not be able to pinpoint what caused your loved one's emotional upheaval or why, but it can help to be aware that certain themes and patterns do tend to come up over and over. Most themes for people with BPD, directly or indirectly, have something to do with invalidation.*

When you can't make your loved one's pain go away, eventually you either withdraw or move in and try to make everything better. Withdrawing causes your loved one to feel more desperate and hopeless. Trying to fix everything causes your loved one to feel helpless and hopeless. Trying to protect your partner from anything that will trigger a painful emotion exhausts you and just doesn't work. So what can you do instead?

*W*hat You Can Do Differently When Your Loved One Is Trapped in an Emotional Whirlpool

Here's the thing about whirlpools and quicksand: Try to jump in and pull someone out and you're likely to get pulled in too. Whatever you do to try to "save" your loved one from her own emotions elicits another emotional reaction, often one that makes *you* overly emotional. So the first thing you can do differently in response to your relative with BPD is to try not to respond from emotion.

1. Ask yourself what emotion you're having and focus on not responding from the emotion. As you saw in Chapter 4, regulating your own emotion is always the first step in responding effectively to someone with BPD. This is true no matter which of the faces of BPD described in Part II you're seeing. But it's paramount when your partner is being pulled down by emotional vulnerability. Let's say your spouse or sibling or best friend is going back and forth between extreme sadness and despair that her life is not different and anger at you. It's only human to have emotional reactions to being attacked. In addition, believing that your loved one might actually lose control of her emotions and the consequences might be dire is frightening. It's these high emotions of your own that can cause you to make frantic attempts to fix things or to withdraw from your loved one. The former, as you've learned, makes it difficult to react wisely and with attention to your partner's experience. This only makes your loved one feel invalidated and may make him attack you further. The latter will make your partner feel abandoned and certainly won't do anything constructive to keep your relationship intact. So, the first thing to do is to regulate your own emotions.

Remember the client I described in Chapter 2 who just kept expressing anger at me no matter what I tried to say and finally exploded, saying that all she'd wanted was to have me help her with one problem and I wasn't doing my job? Honestly, at that moment, I just wanted to stop the session, but instead I got quiet. I got quiet so that I could regulate my own emotions and determine what to do next. When I quit talking, my client quit talking also. Like me, when she got quiet, her emotions came down, and after a few minutes we moved on. Of course, we had used all of the session time with her being upset and angry with me because I just didn't get that reacting to her attacks the way I had was exacerbating the situation.

If you find yourself losing control or at a loss for how to respond to your loved one's emotional outbursts, stop and notice what you're feeling. Follow the steps for regulating your emotion in Chapter 4, noticing your physical sensations, thoughts, and urges. If you add up the observations that your stomach hurts, your chest is tight, your hands are clenched, your forehead is wrinkled, you're frowning, and you have an urge to tell your loved one everything you're thinking about her right now, you will be able to understand that the emotion you are experiencing is anger.

If the ideas for regulating your emotion from Chapter 4 aren't working, try to shift to accepting your emotions in a mindful mode. If you're too overwrought to even observe your own experience, start by staying silent and taking a deep breath. Breathe in and out. It doesn't have to be deep or slow; just focus for a moment on the path of your breath. Focus on having a wise response and not one that is emotional. If you can't bring your emotion down by breathing, try counting something in the room where you are. If you can take a break from the problem at that point, do it. Go and do something that calms your senses, like taking a bath, listening to calming music, sitting outside and watching nature, eating something soothing. The key to using these "skills" is to do them mindfully. Being mindful means putting all of your attention into what you are doing and not thinking about what is happening with your loved one. Your thoughts will inevitably go back to the event that caused you to be emotional or worry about your loved one. When you notice that you are thinking about other things, "grab" your mind and bring it back to what you were doing. Then, when you are less emotional, you can help your loved one.

> Go back to the box on page 75 in Chapter 4 and consider using the skill "opposite action" if you're not succeeding in defusing your own emotions.

People with BPD are regulated externally. This means that they are regulated by things in their environment, and that includes you. If the environment is calming, they will calm. They will be more skillful in a helpful relationship than on their own. The good news is that you can help them regulate their emotions just by regulating your own—a whole different ballgame from *telling* them to control *their* emotions.

A *caveat:* It's easy when being calm to talk to people with BPD in a tone of voice you might use with a child. This is problematic in a couple of ways. First, the already aroused emotions of people with BPD will escalate if they perceive themselves as being treated condescendingly. Who wouldn't? Being patronized evokes a strong reaction in all of us. Second, speaking this way can be tantamount to treating your loved one as if she were fragile when she is not. This will either invalidate her emotions or send the message that she is incapable.

2. Avoid the *don'ts* that invalidate. If your loved one gets more upset when you're only trying to help, ask yourself whether you're following these "rules of engagement" with someone caught in the emotional vortex:

- *Don't say anything* before you try to express some genuine understanding of your loved one's emotional experience. A general rule is to make at least two validating statements ("I understand"; "This is really important to you") before trying to solve the problem. Giving advice, trying to distract her, or telling her "it's not so bad" are all invalidating. Your love and concern won't be heard; all your loved one will hear is that *you don't get how badly she's hurting right now.* To people without BPD, just saying in a nonaccusatory fashion that you don't understand why they're reacting the way they are invites them to talk to you openly to explain. To someone with BPD it will often increase the emotion.

> People with BPD have had it with hearing that their emotions don't make sense to others.

- *Don't try to ask your loved one to be different.* People with BPD are very sensitive to anything that may sound like "Pull yourself up by the bootstraps." Anything you say that includes the word *just* is likely to convey that you think it should be easy for your loved one to change the way she is with a snap of her fingers. Avoid saying things like "Just get out of bed," "Just quit yelling," and "Just change how you're thinking."

- *Don't withhold a solution to the problem if you have it . . . but don't try to "fix" things without asking if your help is wanted.* The reason that "Ask" is a crucial step in the five-step response discussed in Chapter 4 is that intervening and trying to make things better for the person with BPD can devalue his pain. "If you understood how hopeless I am," he may think, "you would not even *try* to solve my life problems." Or it communicates that the person is so out of control that others have to intervene. If you don't ask whether your relative is interested in help from you, you may give the impression of invalidating the intensity of her emotion or validating her incompetence. The time to ask is after you've regulated your own emotions and properly validated those of your loved one; see number 6 below.

- *Don't say anything you don't mean sincerely.* People with BPD aren't fools. And they are acutely sensitive to what others think of them. Several researchers in BPD believe that people with BPD are actually better at reading other people's emotions than the rest of us, especially anger. I have had clients tell me that I was angry at them when I wasn't yet aware that I was. Because of this sensitivity, they can usually detect insincerity without fail. When you talk to your loved one, don't play therapist. Be yourself, don't say anything you don't really mean, and don't use words you wouldn't use in ordinary conversation.

- *Don't say "We need to . . . "; say, "Would it be helpful for you to . . . ?"* One little word can say a lot to your loved one. When emotions are already high, there's nothing more patronizing—

and thus invalidating—than the word *we* when what you're saying presumes that you have the right to speak for both you and your loved one.

3. Find something to validate about the person's *current* emotions. If your loved one is expressing anger, you may well be aware that the anger is secondary to some other emotion. *Do not* tell your loved one that her anger is covering up or allowing her to escape from some other hurt, pain, shame, or other emotion. Instead, validate the anger and then try a little mind reading (see Level 3 validation in Chapter 3) about the other emotion: "You're really angry about work, and that's hard because you know you need to go back tomorrow. I'll bet you're pretty hurt about how she treated you, too. Are you?" Communicate understanding of how painful the person's life is.

4. Validate the person's sense of not being able to control his emotions. You might say something like "Does your anger feel out of control? It must be really uncomfortable." Or "It's really hard to feel out of control" or "I have a hard time when I feel out of control" or "Are you feeling out of control, like anger is just going to consume you? That must be really hard." The point to make at first is not that the person can control his emotions or should be able to control his emotions and not that he is not really out of control. The first thing is to find something you can say that lets your loved one know you get that he's feeling out of control and that being out of control is a painful, scary place.

5. Next, communicate your hope and belief in the person's ability to get in control. This is not to say that your loved one shouldn't be where she is right now but that you have faith in her own capacity to regulate her emotions. This really is cheerleading your loved one. As noted above, it has to be done genuinely and with awareness. If you start telling your loved one that you know she can do this, that she's done it before, and you notice that her emotions are rising or she says, "You don't know what I can do. I can't do it. I've tried everything and I'm tired of trying so hard," back off and go back to validating your loved one's current emotions.

Remind your loved one of times when she has felt like this and gotten through while still validating how hard it is. When she says "I can't stand feeling like this anymore," say "I know it feels like you can't take it. You're a person of incredible strength, and I've seen you make it through times like this before. I have complete faith in your ability to get through this." Asking interested questions is a great alternative to making suggestions that can sound like you are intervening and interfering because you have no faith in your loved one's abilities: "Do you remember when you and Bob broke up? How did you get through it then? I know that was devastating for you, but you made it." Or you might ask, "Can you do something that has been helpful before?"

> I ask my clients to make me the keeper of the hope and to look to me for hope. If you genuinely feel such hope, you can do the same for your loved one.

6. Ask if your loved one would like help in solving whatever problem has caused this pain. As noted above, saying "Here's what you need to do" without finding out first whether your relative wants advice is bound to raise, not lower, emotion. "Ask/assess" is an important step in the five-step response described in Chapter 4. Remember that you might not get a clear answer, however. The person may refuse to participate in this mode of interacting. Emotions may still be too high. As suggested in Chapter 4, whenever a person with BPD answers the question "How can I help?" with something like "You can't help; there's nothing anyone can do," you should go back to validation. Say, "I know it feels that way right now. I don't know if I can help. I am sure willing to try." Don't try to make your loved one problem-solve. You might suggest doing some brainstorming together. But remember that her ability to generate ideas is severely compromised. All of us lose the ability to focus, brainstorm, and choose solutions to our problems when we are emotional. All of the neurochemical processes and changes in our brain chemistry in response to emotions interfere with our ability to problem-solve. So if you start trying to brainstorm and your loved one gives up and says "There is no solution—there's nothing I can do," don't conclude she is being passive or uncooperative. It is often just that the person's emotions are so high that she cannot think of any solutions in this state of mind. In that case you can always suggest coming back to it later.

7. When all else fails, when you can't mind-read, go back to validation. As explained in Chapter 4, the key is to stay aware of your loved one's emotional responses to you during these interactions. If his emotions start intensifying, move back into validating. If they are subsiding, ask how you can help.

When emotions are running high, it's awfully hard not to have your own emotions stirred up, and then you get pulled down into the whirlpool with the person who is struggling with BPD. That's why I've spent so much time in this chapter elaborating on the ideas you read about in Chapter 4 for responding to emotions that feel unbearable to your loved one. Understand that your sister or friend or son is biologically vulnerable to intense, persistent emotion and has learned that these emotions are unacceptable, and you'll stop wasting so much energy trying to get this person to do something that he or she is just not capable of doing right now. Learn and apply the skills described here, and you relieve yourself of an emotional burden as well as create an environment

---

Helping Your Loved One Use Opposite Action

In the same way that you can change an emotional response of your own (see Chapter 4), you can observe your loved one to see if you can identify her emotion and then gently nudge her toward an action that is opposite that emotion. Every emotion has an action urge, something that it makes you want to do. Think about young children and you will see the action of emotions. If they get scared, they'll run from whatever is fearsome. When angry, they attack either physically or verbally. When sad, they withdraw from everyone. If they feel guilty, they will do something to make things better, like apologize. Is your relative's primary emotional state one of increased physiological arousal (like anger or fear) or decreased physiological arousal (like sadness)? If you can't determine the emotion, determine what action urge your loved one has. Then try to get her to do the opposite of the action urge to get the emotion to decrease in intensity or change. Instead of running from something frightening, see if you can suggest a way she could approach it. If she is afraid of applying for jobs because she has been turned down before, tell her you know she's afraid, recognize that she has been turned down, and then say, "You know the only way you are ever going to get that fear to go down is to apply for jobs. I know the thought strikes fear in your soul. I guess the question is 'Do you want your fear to go down?'" If she's sad, opposite action might be to get out of her bedroom and do something that makes her feel competent and in control of her emotions and/or her life.

conducive to your loved one's learning to regulate his or her emotions over time. Remember that your loved one is dysregulated by emotions and then becomes more emotional because the emotions feel so out of control. Remember, also, that there is really no one as critical and blaming of the person with BPD as that person, and you'll find it easier to exercise the compassion you already feel. The next chapter talks about the insidious self-blame that drives people with BPD and how you can deal with it.

"It Was All My Fault"

Laura had been sobbing for hours, begging her husband, Steve, to understand that her sadness was out of control. She wanted him to do something—*anything*—to make the pain stop. Steve had tried everything he could think of to help Laura. He tried soothing her with tea and comfort. Then he shifted into practical mode and tried to "get to the bottom" of what was bothering his wife. It seemed like everything he tried only made Laura more distraught, and soon he found himself begging *her* to help *him* figure out how to make her feel better. Thoroughly drained, Laura eventually left the room to wash her face. When she came back, her tears had dried. As she spoke, her voice shook from the efforts that it took to control herself. "I shouldn't be feeling this way at all, and now I'm hurting you, the person I love most," she said. "I'll be fine. Don't you worry about me for another minute. I'm being a terrible person, and I don't deserve to have you. I don't need to talk about this anymore. It's all right."

More than anything, Steve wanted to believe Laura. But experience told him that it wouldn't be all right and that this scene would be repeated, as it had been for years. He wasn't sure how much more he could take. Sometimes he wanted to shout at Laura that she was lying, that she was self-indulgent, that she lived in some crazy fantasy world where she was at the center of everything. A couple of times he'd actually blurted out his feelings, and the result had been disastrous. Once Laura had drunk half a bottle of gin and then gotten in the car, and it had been sheer luck that he had been able to stop her before she drove off. Another time she had picked up the phone and called her boss at home to tell him she was quitting her job because she was incompetent and out of touch with reality.

The fact that Laura's mood and behavior seem to change so quickly and unpredictably leaves Steve feeling like he has no control, which makes him feel like he can't help her stop feeling so bad. As you read in Chapter 4, it's true that he has no direct control over how bad she feels. It's not true, however, that Laura can't change. But she needs help. She needs people on the outside to help her shut off the self-critical voice she keeps hearing on the inside.

People who have BPD often have periods of time when they beat themselves up, insisting that they are worthless, undeserving, inept. This pattern of behavior is called *self-invalidation*, and it is a learned behavior. All of us learn behavior. If you are brought up in a family where you are told "Quit that crying or I'll give you something to cry about," you will learn to stifle the urge to cry. You may not do this after the first time you hear the statement or the third time, but eventually being told to quit crying and actually stopping crying will become part of your behavior. In situations that make you feel like crying, you will automatically stop yourself from crying. In the case of self-invalidation, a person with BPD, like Laura, will prevent herself from crying by telling herself that there is nothing to cry about, that she should just stop. Or she'll use whatever invalidating words she has learned in her life. In other chapters, we will talk about how emotion can stop automatically, without a thought or a word shutting it down.

If you think of the emotional whirlpool described in Chapter 4 as existing on one end of the spectrum of borderline behavior, self-invalidation is at the opposite end. However, these two patterns most often appear in the same person. Your loved one may get pulled into the emotional vortex as emotion builds on emotion, but as her rawness increases, the emotions become totally overwhelming and then, because she literally cannot stand it anymore, she moves into invalidating her experience. All of a sudden, those emotions that were so strong are irrelevant or don't exist. Or the problems that caused them can be solved with ease. Sometimes those with BPD may minimize their problems because they can't accurately communicate them. Or they might minimize them to protect others, a behavior called *apparent competence* (described in Chapter 8).

Of course, if anyone self-invalidates long enough, those extreme emotions will come back. As Laura beats up on herself and tells herself she is overreacting and should just "get over it," the intensity of the emotions builds. Hopelessness and anger are often the results of self-invalidation. The person with BPD feels hopeless about ever getting better, deciding that she's incompetent and doesn't deserve to live. Anger can be directed at herself for being worthless and incompetent or at others for not recognizing how bad the state of her life really is. As these emotions build, she moves back into emotional vulnerability, as discussed in Chapter 5. Once your loved one is in that state of heightened emotional vulnerability, it's as if she's riding a pendulum, and the momentum is hard to disrupt. She keeps swinging from devastatingly intense emotion to desperate attempts to deny the emotion's validity and back to very strong emotion. If you've witnessed these swings, you know how painful it is to watch and feel helpless to stop the pendulum. You can undoubtedly also easily imagine how agonizing it must be to be the one riding the pendulum.

In the case of Steve and Laura, Laura stops all of her emotion and promises Steve that she will not lose control again. She punishes herself for making problems in the family. She sets unrealistic goals, like "I'll never be upset again." It's important to understand that she means it. She is making a real promise not to get into the position of being so emotionally out of control. The problem is that for Laura this promise is impossible to keep. Emotions grow through the cracks in her self-invalidation. Because she is judging herself and setting unrealistic expectations for herself ("I just won't have emotions"), she first begins to feel upset with herself about her own behavior. As she tells herself she is a terrible partner, an awful person, and so forth, her guilt, shame, and despair build. Over time, these emotions build back into emotional vulnerability, and then she plunges back into the abyss of emotion. Maybe your loved one with BPD doesn't look exactly like Laura in this not-very-detailed example. But she may manifest self-invalidation in some more subtle way. Self-invalidation can take the form of three different behavioral patterns:

Some people invalidate their own emotional experiences even when their reactions are justifiable. You just heard Laura say she shouldn't be having the emotions she was having. Maybe she was right: if she was suffering deep distress over having lost a ballpoint pen, her emotions would certainly seem to be out of proportion to the circumstances. But what if her beloved cat had just died? In that case her emotional response might have been perfectly valid. The problem with self-invalidation in BPD is that the person is quite likely to insist his emotions are invalid when anyone else would believe they were perfectly justifiable. People who are self-invalidating might, for example, tell themselves that they should not be experiencing frustration with a coworker when anyone else would feel frustrated in the same circumstances. When they suffer a loss, they deny the experience of sadness. They inhibit the experience of the emotions.

You might not actually see this process going on. But one thing you might be able to observe is your loved one appearing to be calm. In fact, she may be calm because she is suppressing the emotions, negating them. In that case your loved one is attempting to just turn off the emotions with force of will. She is likely to have learned to try this earlier in life, but we know from research that when anyone suppresses emotions over time, they tend to rebound. And when they do come back, they come up unexpectedly and strongly.

Invalidating their own emotions, justifiable and otherwise, can trigger a variety of responses that create more pain and difficulty, both for those with BPD and for their loved ones. When he has emotions, your loved one may respond to them with self-criticism and shame. Shame becomes its own intense emotion, which he then criticizes and thus increases the feeling of shame. We call shame "the mortal enemy" of people with BPD, and it's the predominant problem emotion for them. It is highly correlated with suicide, self-harm, and other impulsive behaviors. Shame builds very quickly and cuts people off from others. Just think about how a person feeling intense shame behaves: She will sit with her head down and not engage. This makes her feel more disconnected, more shameful, and ultimately leads to more problematic behaviors.

> Shame is mortal enemy number one for people with BPD. Hopelessness is mortal enemy number two.

Your loved one might also respond to invalidating his own emotions by absorbing all the painful events of the world—his own and those that have stricken others. The message heard so often by people with BPD that their pain is unacceptable and unreal echoes so loudly in their heads that they tend to look for evidence to confirm their lack of worth. Absorbing painful events is a way of gathering information about why they really don't deserve to exist. They think they cause all of the painful events or, like in the case of 9/11, don't think they deserve to exist when others suffered. Even though they usually don't recognize it as such, the result is often hopelessness, as mentioned in Chapter 5. Because it can feed suicidal thoughts, hopelessness is mortal enemy number two for those with BPD.

Some people don't trust their own emotional responses to situations. People with BPD who are engaged in self-invalidation believe they are so deficient that they don't experience emotions as others do. Has your loved one ever said, in the thick of some situation that would stimulate an emotion in most people, "I don't know how I am supposed to feel"? Has she ever asked you, "How do *you* think I should feel about this?" Many of us have expressed such doubts when we've felt conflicting emotions or when we've had reason to be concerned that we might be overreacting. In those cases we're usually trying to work through our feelings in our own mind, or we're asking for a reality check from someone we trust. Those with BPD, however, doubt their own emotional experience to such a degree that some come to rely entirely on external input to define their internal experience. Their self-doubt about their internal experience can even hinder their ability to name their emotions in the first place. Self-invalidation leads them to think something like "What I feel is wrong, pathological, and so crazy that I don't even know what it is."

Finally, people with BPD are often overly perfectionistic. This is a somewhat paradoxical behavior pattern that may really throw you. Your loved one may set unrealistically high goals and standards for herself. In anyone else, aspiring to achievements that seem pretty clearly out of reach as conceived might appear to be grandiose. Someone who thinks he can succeed via a single gigantic leap rather than through lots of small steps might be viewed as lacking humility. But for the person with BPD these unrealistic aspirations represent the opposite. To try to change their own behavior, people with BPD will focus on punishing themselves—setting unattainable goals and then declaring themselves worthless, *as they expected*, when those lofty aspirations prove out of reach.

Maybe you've seen your loved one struggling with knowing how to change his behavior slowly, over time, and with rewards. Instead of saying, "I want to get a job in the advertising industry—that is my goal—so I will start by working as a receptionist in the company," he says, "I want to be in advertising. I am going to apply for Director of Marketing. If I don't get the job, it's because I am stupid and don't deserve a good job." And, of course, because he has no experience, he doesn't get the job as Director of Marketing. Then he begins to berate himself: He is incapable, worthless, and hopeless. Often someone caught in this trap tells himself that things will never get any better and that everyone else will be better off if he kills himself. At the least, this experience of "failure" leaves the person unwilling to try new things out of fear of "failing" again. Ultimately, he may avoid taking the risks that would help him feel competent. Cindy was a woman who had enormous potential. She had graduated at the top of her high school class and had begun college. Then she fell in love and quit school to raise her family. Over the years, she had multiple hospitalizations and began to drink daily. People would tell her that she should get out, get a job, volunteer—anything to make herself feel better. Cindy would talk about how she was going to go back to school and finish her social work degree. Everyone knew that Cindy would gain momentum after she started school and realized that she could pass the classes. However, in spite of her talk, Cindy never began a class. Cindy did not think she could pass. She saw herself as stupid and broken. She felt so much shame about being less than capable that she never enrolled in the program. Her shame kept her from doing something that would have built some mastery, made her feel better about herself, and ultimately decreased the shame.

Setting unreasonable goals and then not meeting them is something often seen with impulsive behaviors like substance abuse. Right after using, the person with BPD will adamantly assert, "I am through with drugs. I am not going to use them ever again. I don't need any help with quitting, because I just quit." She uses a "will power" model of stopping using drugs, one that was learned from a "pull yourself up by the bootstraps" lesson in life. Ultimately, this person uses again. Then her guilt and shame increase. She begins to punish herself for having used. She is full of self-blame and criticism. Her self-loathing skyrockets. She tries to kill herself because she doesn't deserve to live.

Self-harm is another impulsive behavior about which people with BPD become unrealistic. If your loved one cuts herself, she'll tell you that she is never going to cut again and then refuse to talk about it. If your loved one has said things like this, how have you interpreted the behavior? It's easy to fall prey to the assumption that your loved one is trying to get you to quit bugging her or make you beg for more information. Or maybe you've concluded that she doesn't want to talk about cutting just because it's unpleasant. Sometimes the reality is that in that moment she does not believe she will cut again. Then, when she has an urge, she crashes.

*H*ow to Respond to Self-Invalidation

Earlier I said that Laura probably wouldn't be fine and unless she got help to turn off her self-invalidation the same scene would probably keep playing out between her and Steve. So how do you change someone's self-invalidating behavior? You can change the behaviors of others by changing your own behavior to some extent. As noted in Chapter 5, those with BPD are regulated externally, which means you can certainly exert some influence. But your loved one may need professional help to change his or her behavior in other contexts. And remember that the self-invalidation and emotional vulnerability will still be there. With that in mind, here are some suggestions.

Validate the Emotions and the Experience, Not the Self-Invalidation

What do we typically do when those we love put themselves down? We say it isn't so—they're not stupid, bad, clumsy, pushy, or whatever negative label they've applied to themselves. It's really painful to hear someone we care about talk about being worthless, stupid, undeserving, and so forth. So our immediate reaction is to counter the statement by negating it. Your spouse says, "I should have been able to handle that situation—I am totally stupid," and your instinctive desire is to say "You're *not* stupid." We think that's the kind of support and reassurance our loved ones want from us, and in the absence of BPD we may be exactly right. When your loved one has BPD, though, you'll need to apply a lot of patience and be prepared to do some adept validating. The key is to validate your loved one's experiences and emotions without validating the self-invalidation.

This is a corollary of the "rule" you read in Chapter 3 never to validate the invalid. It may sound a little like double-talk, but if you simply say "You're *not* stupid" to your loved one's assertion that she is, you're invalidating her emotional experience even though you may believe you're invalidating only a false conclusion she's drawn about herself.

What you say will be viewed as your trying to change your loved one's emotions by arguing that they aren't accurate. Your loved one won't hear that she's worthy and loved. She's saying she *feels* stupid, and to her you're saying she *shouldn't* feel that way: that her emotions are untrustworthy, invalid, or just plain wrong. You're only confirming what she's been hearing for her whole life!

What you have to learn to do is to separate your reaction to your loved one's experience from your reaction to the conclusion she has drawn from feeling her emotions. So, tell her that you know she has had a difficult time, the situation was hard, and you know she feels stupid. Then, depending on the situation, you might offer to help her solve the problem, or you might offer reassurance that she is not stupid at that point. If you notice that her emotions are on the rise, back down and go back to validating.

The *Right* Way to Counter Self-Invalidation

1. *Validate the person's experience*: She's had a tough time, the situation was difficult, things didn't turn out as expected, she doesn't know what to do next.

2. *Validate the person's emotions*: You know she *feels* stupid, she *feels* like a failure, she *feels* like things will never get better, she *feels* ashamed and/or hopeless.

3. *Offer to help solve the problem or reassure her that her conclusions about herself are inaccurate—if her emotions seem to be waning.*

4. *If you try Step 3 and notice the person's emotions building again, return to validation.*

Encourage Slow Change

It's important for people with BPD to learn to tolerate gradual changes in behavior and slowly attain goals and expectations. We call slow change "shaping." By definition, shaping is gradual approximation to a goal. The key is to allow change in increments and reinforce each step. I can't say that persuading people with BPD to allow slow change and to

reward themselves for new behavior instead of trying to punish themselves into new behavior is easy. The key is to find the small steps to
validate. Let's go back to Cindy. Cindy believes the only thing that
counts is being in school and making As, and the fact that she believes
herself incapable of achieving this keeps her from even trying to enroll
in a class. But one day she goes online and looks at a college site. Her
friends and relatives could help her by reinforcing that effort. They
might say, "That's great—I remember getting so excited about college
once I started to look at all the different things each one has to offer" or
"Aren't the college websites great? You can really dig into the area you're
interested in and get details you might not have gotten from one of the
printed college guides." The point is to be mindful only of what is happening *now* and not to focus on the goal. So reinforcing what Cindy
might be getting out of accom-
plishing this step instead of how
this step is getting her closer to
the ultimate goal may help deter
her from self-invalidation. This
is easier to do with action-
oriented goals like Cindy's or
one such as cleaning out the garage than with other behaviors. With
self-invalidation specifically, you might try noticing and reinforcing a
time when the person with BPD does not self-invalidate or stops in the
middle of self-invalidation.

> When reinforcing incremental
> steps to encourage slow change,
> it's essential to be genuine.
> Any hint of patronization will
> reinforce self-invalidation.

Here are some guidelines to follow:

- *Never negate your loved one's goals.* Even if you know your loved
one can't possibly meet these goals, tell yourself that it's not your place
to tell him whether he can achieve a goal. This can be really tough
when the fallout of your loved one's failed efforts has been an imposition
on you; the last thing you may want is to allow him to keep going off
in "crazy" directions instead of developing competence through success.
To resist the instinct to tell him he's "dreaming," make yourself find a
small piece that you can concentrate on. If he wants to quit drugs forever and you don't believe there's any way he can, tell him to know that
he can stay off drugs today. If she wants to be president of a software
firm, validate that she enjoys computers. If you truly don't believe the
goal is attainable, don't lie. Find something else to validate.

- *Steer your loved one toward breaking down the goal into many little achievable steps.* Small, potentially achievable steps breed success. But they also allow time to review, reconsider, and regroup. If your loved one starts making gradual progress toward a larger goal, the confidence built by these little successes can serve as armor against the instinctive reaction that any little failure is a reflection of "the big failure" of the person himself. With a little breathing room in between steps, the person also has the luxury of thinking things over—"I did okay at *this*," but I'm not enjoying [or I'm having trouble with] *that*, and I'd have to be good at *that* to reach my final destination." Even better, the person might discover something else he really is good at that suggests a new end goal. Meanwhile, *you* haven't invalidated what your loved one wants in his life.

I had a client once who had dropped out of high school because she had missed too many days. Then her drinking and her cutting increased and she had been very suicidal for about 12 years. While in treatment with me, she decided that she wanted to go to medical school. I didn't tell her how skeptical I was that a 30-year-old with no high school diploma and many years of being out of control could actually get through medical school. Instead, I worked with her to make a list of everything she needed to get to medical school. We broke it down to small, achievable goals and had her begin. As she worked on her GED, we realized that she needed even smaller goals, so we made weekly study goals. Then we set a schedule for what she was going to do each weekend to reward herself for meeting her weekly goals.

Of course, there were moments when she wanted to give up. She would have a hard week with her studies and would want to quit. She would tell me that she was dumb, that she was crazy, that she couldn't do it. I would tell her that I didn't actually know for a fact that she could do it, but that I believed in her. I would assure her that we all have moments in school when we don't feel so smart. Ultimately, she went to phlebotomy school and is in the medical profession. She realized over time that medical school was not really an option. What she really learned, though, was how to tolerate emotions without self-invalidating and how to have small, achievable, reinforceable goals.

Help Your Loved One Check the Facts

Self-invalidating people have to learn to tolerate their own emotional experiences. It's important to remember that what is precipitating the self-criticism is often emotion. The emotion fires, the emotion is difficult, and the person with BPD invalidates the emotion as wrong, bad, and so forth. When something bad happens to people with BPD, as it happens to all of us, they begin to believe that bad things happen to them because they are bad. When this is the case, it's often useful to help your loved one check the facts. This does *not* mean telling him that bad things happen to all of us. It is about looking at the facts of the situation. Remember these guidelines:

- *Ask the person to say exactly what happened without adding to it.* So, it's not "I'm so stupid and the tire blew on the interstate. I don't deserve to be able to go out with friends." It is "I was driving down the interstate. It was 10 o'clock at night. I had been to dinner with friends. My tire blew out on the interstate."

- *Now ask what emotion the person was having at the time.* My guess, in the case of the tire blowout, is that it was probably fear.

- *Then validate the emotion.* Any of us would have some anxiety if we blew a tire out at night. Especially if we are women. That is a dangerous situation.

- *Encourage the person to describe the behavior in the moment without generalizing to an interpretation of something larger (who he is as a person, how others feel about him, etc).* Even after you've validated the emotion, most people with BPD will immediately tell you how it's their fault that the event occurred. The fact is, the car owner *could* have something to do with a tire blowing. It could be that the tires are old and worn and the last time he had the oil changed he was told he needed new tires but put it off. It could be that he had a nail in his tire that he needed to have removed and he had not done so. In these cases, allow your loved one to own the behavior but not to leap from not getting the tire fixed to being bad or incapable. You can do this by sticking to the facts yourself. You might say something like "Okay, so you knew that you needed to get the nail out of the tire. We'll agree that next time you will have that done, right?"

- *Be a broken record—and don't be lured into arguing the accuracy of your loved one's self-criticism.* If your loved one returns to how he's bad, repeat that he knew he should fix the tire, but don't argue for or against his being a stupid person.

Dealing with Shame

To respond appropriately to a person with BPD, you must know something about shame. Our culture has little understanding of shame. I often hear therapists say that no one should experience shame under any circumstances, yet shame evolved to keep us alive. For our tribal ancestors it was imperative to avoid doing anything that would get them kicked out of the tribe. Being exiled inevitably meant death, from starvation, exposure, or predation. Shame, by urging us to keep our behaviors secret, prevented individuals from revealing anything to the rest of the tribe that would get them ejected.

When I worked with women in prison, I found that they felt a lot of shame and guilt (emotions that occur when we violate our own values) over their crimes. I used to tell them that if they were released from prison, they should use their shame to keep them from telling people who didn't know them who they were and/or what they had done. If they went to a neighborhood party as newcomers and revealed their criminal behavior and imprisonment, they'd be ostracized. They could instead use their shame to keep them from telling their secrets unnecessarily.

The problem is that most of the time our shame isn't justified. The secrets we could tell generally won't get us kicked out of the tribe. For example, I love reality television. I used to not tell anyone that I watched certain shows because I was ashamed of it. I thought there was really something wrong with me for watching these shows. Finally I realized that my shame wasn't justified. Most people weren't going to reject me if they were talking about reality TV and I said I watched it.

Odds are your loved one often experiences high levels of shame. Sometimes it's easy to think that people who repeatedly engage in behaviors that are so problematic would not feel shame and guilt about their mistakes. Think about how your loved one acts when you try to talk about certain subjects. If he stays silent, looks down, or changes the subject, there's a good chance he's feeling shame. The shame is compounded when the person with BPD inevitably criticizes his own behavior, his emotions, and even his shame. This, of course compounds all of the emotions and drags the person back into the emotional vortex.

The only way to get the shame to subside is to get your loved one to talk about what is causing the shame. She has to talk about whatever it is over and over while making eye contact to get the shame to go down. If she is talking to you, you must make sure you don't do anything that could be interpreted as rejection. So, you can't look away from her or laugh at what she says. Her brain has to learn that she is not being "kicked out of her tribe" for her behaviors or emotions. Over time, her shame will come down, but how much time it will take and whether this exposure to shame can be instigated by you or should be done by a therapist depends on the level of shame and the behavior that precipitates it. Victims of abuse, for example, really need the help of a therapist to overcome shame.

When I was treating my reality television show shame, I made myself join in conversations about the popular shows. I would make eye contact with whoever was in the conversation, and I worked up to a point where I could say proudly, "I LOVE reality television." When I did, my shame diminished.

For your loved one, the situation that is firing the shame is often much more life altering than reality television. People with BPD typically have had problems in the past and have engaged in behaviors that make them feel like there is something fundamentally broken or wrong with them. Whenever a memory of the past comes up or when they encounter a situation in the present that was like a past experience, shame begins to fire again. The problem is that shame is generalizing from past to present experiences and from context to context. Again, shame from trauma is best treated by therapists, but you can still help with shame in the present. The important principle for you is to get the person to talk about whatever is triggering the *current* shame. The person should talk about it over and over until the shame diminishes. For example: Your loved one does apply for the job and interviews but does not get the job. She does not want to tell you about it because of shame. Ask her to tell you about the interview and to tell you that she did not get the job. If you can, get her to talk about it over and over. If your loved one says, "I am stupid for not knowing this, but ... " ask her to repeat the statement without the invalidation at the beginning. If your sister wants to tell you something but says, "I can't talk about it. It's too bad. I humiliated myself," you say, "Tell me about it. The only way you're going to come to grips with it is if you do tell me over and over until it's not so humiliating."

Shame in particular and self-invalidation in general may be deeply ingrained in those with BPD, and they take time to tackle. But making the effort is worthwhile because self-invalidation usually leaves people feeling helpless when they are not and don't need to be. If your relative has a history of self-invalidation, she may lack the skills and confidence to problem-solve, and you may see this deficit take shape as what we call *active passivity*, where she demands that you fix her problems for her. Chapter 7 discusses this next manifestation of BPD.

How to Help Your Loved One Overcome Shame

1. Notice when shame comes into the picture. This is most often indicated by the person's looking away or suddenly changing the topic of conversation ("Did you get a haircut?").

2. Don't remove the cue. If you're talking about what happened during the day and your loved one stops making eye contact, don't stop talking about what happened.

3. Don't reinforce shame. Don't communicate that she should feel shame (don't say, "Wow, that really was a stupid response").

4. Don't move on until shame goes down. If your loved one knows that you are trying not to reinforce shame, say, "Are you still thinking there's something wrong with you?" If your loved one does not know that you are trying not to reinforce shame, make sure you keep talking about the topic until he or she stops trying to look away or change the subject.

5. Then reinforce the person or allow the topic to change.

"You Have to Fix This for Me!"

Have you ever had a conversation that looked like this?

> PAUL: I need you to go to the bank for me. My checking account is all screwed up.
>
> SUSAN: Paul, I don't have time to go for you. I have a meeting, and the kids have parent–teacher conferences today.
>
> PAUL: But I can't do it. I can't figure out what I did wrong. I need you to take care of this. If you cared about me, you'd do it.
>
> SUSAN: I just really don't have time.
>
> PAUL: (*voice getting louder and higher*) I CAN'T DO IT. YOU NEED TO GO TO THE BANK OR I'LL JUST OVERDRAW THE ACCOUNT.

Of course, in this scenario, Susan ultimately felt like she did not have a choice but to go to the bank. She was afraid of the consequences of the account being overdrawn, and she believed that Paul couldn't accomplish the banking on his own. She felt frustrated with Paul, the situation, and herself because she knew that by going to the bank she was communicating to Paul that she agreed that he was somehow incapable of taking care of the banking.

If your loved one has a history of acting similarly to Paul, you're probably increasingly frustrated. Maybe you've tried to show your sister or son how to handle the problem he or she keeps bringing to you, but your coaching doesn't seem to take. Or you'd generally be willing to assist with problems that you know are complicated for anyone to tackle alone ... if only your relative would ask nicely instead of demanding heatedly. You could be lying awake at night trying to figure out how someone so smart seems to turn into a helpless child when least expected. At times you might agonize over whether this person you care about is just taking advantage of you to spare herself some effort.

People who behave like Paul are engaging in what we call *active-passivity*. In this state, your relative is adopting a passive problem-solving style. For somewhat complicated reasons, your loved one feels incapable of solving a problem at hand and therefore turns to you to get the job done. Those with BPD do not do this to spare themselves effort, to get attention, or to abdicate responsibility. They do not feel good about conducting their lives this way. Quite the contrary, in fact. Unfortunately, active-passivity can be very alienating. Like Susan, you undoubtedly have a long list of obligations of your own to fulfill. Like Susan, you might often feel torn: Should you try to squeeze in this additional task just to spare yourself the potential fallout of a bigger problem if this one goes unsolved? Or should you "stand up for your rights" and insist that your partner take responsibility (and then keep your fingers crossed)? If you accede to your loved one's requests, your resentment may grow ... and so will your relative's shame. If you decline, you may feel wracked with self-doubt and guilt ("Was I being unfair and unloving?") along with worry, and your loved one may feel more and more desperate and anxious. Where active-passivity is a pattern, it's crucial that you gain an understanding of what's at work. Otherwise this behavior can drive a wedge between you and the person you care about that may be difficult to remove.

*W*hy Can't People with BPD Solve Their Own Problems?

This is the question that can keep you up at night because active-passivity may seem quite paradoxical. People with BPD are just as likely to be innately intelligent as anyone else, so why do they seem like they lack fundamental problem-solving skills? Or maybe you know your loved one actually does have the skills and knowledge to solve a particular problem, so why is he convinced that he can't do it? Sometimes you haven't heard a word about a certain problem until just now; how, then, did your loved one get so desperate to solve it that she's willing to make wildly unreasonable demands of you? For people in Paul's dilemma, two issues could be causing trouble: that they don't know how to solve problems generally (or specifically) and/or that they don't have the confidence to carry out problem solving.

Lack of Problem-Solving Skills

Most people have problem-solving skills, and we use them all the time without labeling the actions we're taking as problem solving. For instance, suppose you are being asked to lead a project at work. You make an assessment: What are your objectives? What do you need? What are the solutions that you can implement (brainstorming)? Which are the best options? What is the timeline for your solutions? What could stop you from meeting your goals? When you answer these questions, you're using problem-solving skills.

You may not believe it, because your loved one with BPD may be capable of handling pretty complex problems in some other arenas, or because your loved one may sometimes convince you that she can "handle it" even when she cannot (a problem known as *apparent competence* and discussed in Chapter 8), but many people with BPD simply haven't learned the skills of problem solving.

How can this be? you're probably asking. Many people seem to acquire the skills of problem solving as naturally as they learn to get out of bed and get going in the morning. Some children may intuit how to come up with and apply solutions. And some people who are very creative use parts of problem-solving strategies just because they are "big picture" people who can look at a problem and brainstorm many possible solutions. Because problem solving is critical to our survival from the moment we are born, some schools are recognizing its importance and actively teaching step-by-step problem solving so that kids not born with an innate knack for it build the skills at a young age.

Problem-solving skills elude people with BPD for the same fundamental reasons that a lot of other BPD-related behaviors arise: emotional dysregulation and invalidation. To put it simply, high emotion often interferes with cognitive abilities. When we say we want to be able to consider a problem with a "clear head," we usually mean with a mind that isn't being bombarded by the action urges of intense emotion. (When you're enraged or terrified, can you quickly and confidently list and analyze your options for responding to someone who has just beaten a puppy or snatched your purse?) Emotional dysregulation can cause cognitive dysfunction, as described in Chapter 1. People who have been highly vulnerable to their emotions throughout life have therefore racked up a lot less experience with successful problem solving; their minds were occupied elsewhere, and they just didn't have the chance to learn what works and what doesn't. More often than not, in fact, their emotions may have led them only to what *doesn't* work.

> In some cases, a person's emotion about the problem at hand—usually anxiety—is so high that she ignores the problem in an attempt to avoid the emotional discomfort, until the problem becomes so huge that it really does require intervention by someone else. That person may often be you.

Then there are the ways that an invalidating environment can interfere with learning problem solving. People with BPD can be denied the experience of effectively solving problems because of others' reactions to their dysregulated emotion or even because others in the family also suffered from emotion dysregulation. In many cases, both factors might be involved.

Imagine an emotionally vulnerable child who is distraught over a common childhood event, such as breaking or losing a favorite toy or being bullied or teased. That child could be taught various ways to deal with the problem—repairing the toy or conducting a systematic search for it; enlisting the aid of an authoritative adult to deal with the meanness of peers or finding a way through hurt feelings. But if the adults in the child's life find the child's emotions intolerable or unacceptable, they might prematurely rush to the rescue to "help" the child. They might scold the child for her reactions ("Quit crying over nothing!"), diverting the child's attention from solving the problem at hand to desperately trying to control emotions she doesn't know how to control. Some might have very rigid problem-solving styles of their own and communicate that there is only one solution to any given problem and that "the" solution must be found, denying the child the opportunity to brainstorm, analyze, and test various solutions to find what works best. In some environments, creative solutions to problems may be punished and family members may be told that they are "crazy" for thinking they can do something or that they will never accomplish it. In cases like these, children learn that it's best to pretend nothing's wrong; or that creativity is not an asset; or that what's expected of them is to sit back and let others solve their problems. They then arrive at adulthood without fully developed problem-solving skills.

In an interesting twist on the role of emotions, some childhood environments actually reinforce children for escalating their emotions. Children are ignored when they ask quietly or politely and with little emotion. What happens when a child is not heard? The child increases the pitch and volume of the request. If it continues to be ignored, the child will continue to increase the intensity of the demand. If, while the child is loud, not skillful at getting what he or she wants, or demanding in voice tone, the environment gives him what he wants, the child learns that increased volume, pitch, and harsh voice tone get him what he needs. Over time, the child evolves into a person who automatically (meaning without thinking) uses a loud, demanding voice to ask people for help.

Lack of Confidence

To launch into problem solving on autopilot as many adults do requires not just skill but also self-confidence. Some people with BPD do possess at least partially developed problem-solving skills. But—*and this happens often with BPD*—even when they have some idea of how to solve the problem, they have no sense that they can do what is needed to solve the problem. Maybe they grew up in an environment that invalidated every unsuccessful effort; "winning" was everything. Maybe it was just that no one paid enough attention to the outcomes of the child's efforts, figuring it was enough that the child had obviously tried, and when things didn't work out, well, "That's life." Experiences like this could leave a child whose emotional experience of disappointment or shame was more intense than average feeling like a "loser" who is better off sparing himself the pain of failure. They could also leave the child without the experience of regrouping, learning from mistakes, and developing mental resilience and creativity.

It's possible that your loved one once knew something about problem solving, but the skills didn't harden into new behaviors because when she tried solving problems she "failed." Sometimes the problem got worse or wasn't solved. If problem solving failed and others criticized the child for trying to solve problems and "getting it wrong," the child would lack confidence and passivity could develop. The person could end up never developing the belief that she can solve her own problems.

What replaces this confidence is an unwavering belief that YOU can solve the problem. People with BPD will in these cases push really hard to get you to solve their problems for them.

*A*re Interpersonal Skills an Issue?

The person you love who has BPD may very well be dealing with another obstacle when it comes to problem solving: a lack of interpersonal skills. As you read in Chapter 1, "interpersonal chaos" is one of the five areas of dysregulation affecting people with BPD. Theoretically, difficulties in knowing how to get along with others could hinder problem solving from a number of angles.

First, if your loved one had problems communicating with others due to emotional dysregulation as a child, he may not have had much success in soliciting constructive problem-solving aid from adults. This is the route by which interpersonal problems could leave an adult with BPD with undeveloped problem-solving skills.

Second, if your relative has rocky relationships with lots of people—perhaps even as a result of poor decision making regarding problems that need to be solved—she may try to avoid problems altogether when they arise, for fear of arousing someone's ire with her "mistakes." People with BPD don't avoid problems just because they want to escape the emotions the problems evoke but also because they're afraid of the interpersonal consequences of "getting it wrong again."

Finally there is the way your loved one requests help—from you and anyone else he has started to rely on. As mentioned above, an adult who learned as a child that the squeaky-wheel approach was the only way to get help with a problem is likely to be loud, strident, and demanding today too when he's stuck—not because he's a bully but because he simply doesn't know any other way. Unfortunately, no one feels particularly magnanimous in the face of forceful demands. You've read stories elsewhere in this book that illustrate how hard it is even for trained therapists to remain open and compassionate. When I have a client who calls me unexpectedly and immediately begins to insist that I "fix her life," and then gets angry and aggressive when I try to apply the five-step response method from Chapter 4, it sometimes takes everything I've got to remain calm and helpful. (Remember how I described the time when the only thing that got us back to a place where we could look at a client's problem objectively was my getting quiet and encouraging her to do the same?)

If you find yourself aggravated in the face of such demands from a loved one, it might help to know what's usually behind this behavior. Besides possibly believing it's the only way to be heard, a person who demands help may very well be operating from high anxiety. People who are convinced that they can't solve a problem, and believe the problem must be solved, naturally feel a lot of anxiety or fear.

Think about fear for a minute: it creates energy, doesn't it? Fear usually serves to make people avoid the thing that causes the fear: you run from snakes, avoid spider webs, don't apply for jobs you are afraid you won't get. Fear has been instrumental in the survival of the human race. If we didn't have fear, we wouldn't have run from the man-eating tigers. Unfortunately, high levels of fear or anxiety interfere with the brain's ability to sort through information and devise new solutions. So, when fear/anxiety rises in your loved one, problem solving—which may already be challenged—decreases. The physiological energy created by the fear/anxiety is still there, but it translates into the manner that your relative takes while asking you to help. What under normal levels of arousal might be "I could really use your help" turns under high anxiety into "Look, you've just got to help me."

> People with BPD aren't trying to evade responsibility for problem solving when they demand that you step in. In that moment, they **are** trying to solve their problems. They're doing it by accessing help from you.

Not all active-passivity takes the form of insistent demands. Some people with BPD instead adopt a helpless stance. If your loved one does this, you may find it just as aggravating if you believe it's not entirely genuine or you're being *guilt-tripped* into being sympathetic. So again, it's important to know what's really going on. Namely, shame is often what is driving your loved one to act helpless. If the person with BPD asks for your help in a quiet, bashful (and sometimes childlike) manner, looking down at the floor, it could be that the active-passivity is driven by shame. People with BPD don't feel good about lacking the ability or confidence to solve their own problems. And the shame they feel may very well have been reinforced over time by their environment and their own tendency toward self-invalidation (see Chapter 6). It could also be that helplessness has been reinforced in your loved one because when she has been helpless before, the environment solved her problems.

It's hard to feel like you're on call to rescue another adult from her own problems—sometimes ordinary, other times extraordinary—especially when the way your loved one asks for help often makes you want to say no. We all know that this interpersonal style pushes people away and makes them less likely, over time, to help. But when you understand that the person you care about may not have had the same opportunity as others to learn to problem-solve, may have been taught not to believe in herself, and may not have the communication skills necessary to ask for help appropriately today, you might be inclined to respond differently to active-passivity. If you do, you will in the process be giving your loved one a chance at remedial skill building that will gradually improve her problem-solving acumen in the future.

*D*on't Confuse Active-Passivity with Passive Aggression

Hannah agreed to host a baby shower for your sister, Bethany. But she procrastinates on the planning, doesn't talk to a baker, forgets to send out invitations, and right before the shower she calls you. Totally distressed, she says she can't do it and the shower needs to be canceled. To keep the shower from being a total disaster, you intervene, get a cake, call people and invite them, and the shower comes off beautifully. You are really angry, however, and as you grumble to yourself, you think, "She's so passive–aggressive."

Think about that. What does that mean? *Passive–aggressive* is an old-fashioned term that has no real meaning. In its day it was considered a "defense mechanism" or a means of reducing anxiety through unconscious behavior. But today it's become a catchall term in the vernacular intended to mean, roughly, "You wanted what ultimately happened to happen, but you didn't want to admit it or take responsibility for wanting that outcome." But would you think in this situation that Hannah had intentionally done this to you? Did she plan to dump the shower in your lap at the last moment? I believe that she probably wanted to host the shower and wanted it to go well. She couldn't get things together

Problem-Solving Steps

If you do problem solving somewhat automatically, you might not be conscious that in the process you're performing the following steps. But if you look at problem solving this way, you might be able to zero in on where your loved one has the greatest difficulty. Then you can use the seven-step response from Chapter 5 to pay particular attention to the step your loved one tends to be least skilled at.

1. **Define the problem**: What are you trying to solve here? What are your goals?

2. **Analyze the problem**: What are the facts about the problem and/or the problem situation?

3. **Generate solutions**: Purely brainstorm. Don't exclude any ideas because they are ridiculous or unrealistic.

4. **Choose a solution**: Narrow down the solutions to the one you think will best get you to your goal, will solve the problem, and is the most realistic to implement.

5. **Troubleshoot the solution**: What could get in the way of achieving the goal? How will you overcome these obstacles?

6. **Put the solution into action**: Try the solution.

7. **Evaluate the solution**: Did it work? If not, choose another solution from the "generate solutions" list and implement it.

and probably put off making arrangements because anxiety interfered with her completing tasks. The next thing she knew, it was time for the shower and she panicked. She really could have canceled the shower, but she believed you could pull it off. And, of course, you did.

Unfortunately, many people who care about someone with BPD think they are being "passive–aggressive" whenever they need to be rescued from a problem.

In fact, we believe that she is not doing anything deliberately. What we believe happened with the shower is that Hannah's style of solving problems is very passive. She doesn't actively attack problems. She probably avoids them. When she begins to try to engage in problem-solving behaviors (getting invitations, talking to the baker, making plans), her emotions go up and her ability to function goes down. Inevitably, she crashes. She may just cancel the shower, but more likely she will behave in a way (either aggressively, "You got me into this—now you need to help me," or passively, "I just can't do this. It's too much for me") that elicits helping behavior from others. So you bail her out by solving the problem. The trouble is, this won't "teach her a lesson" as it might with someone else. Because Hannah has BPD, being bailed out will just make her feel more ashamed than she already did when she couldn't seem to get the shower set up. The fact that you could make a shower happen in 24 hours only reinforces her sense of inadequacy. She hasn't learned anything about problem solving, she'll be more "gun-shy" in the face of the next obligation, and she'll probably invalidate herself to the point where her emotions prevent her from even beginning the steps of problem solving anytime she has a job to do. Hannah's main learning in the situation was that you can solve problems and she can't.

You're not obligated to be your loved one's life coach. No one would tell you it's your job to teach her problem-solving strategies. But if you respond differently to her pleas or demands for help, she might have the chance to start learning them on her own.

How to Respond to Active-Passivity

Carmela doesn't think she's capable of solving her life problems. At the moment, the biggest problem before her is getting her own apartment. So she works hard at getting you to solve it for her. You have other things of importance to work on, and you want her to get an apartment for herself. You don't think that sounds so hard, but she insists she can't do it. She calls and calls. She won't do anything she needs to do to find an apartment, not even read the classifieds to find some good candidates. Now she is about to lose her current living situation and she is still without a new place to live. Either you have to intervene or she will be homeless. You're angry at her for putting you in this position. But she's your daughter and you care about her. You don't want her to be without a residence. And you don't want to have to deal with having her move back home. So you go out, find an apartment for her, and cosign the lease agreement. You wonder how much longer this 28-year-old is going to be so dependent on you and when you're going to have some time for yourself.

To figure out how to respond to active-passivity, you have to start by asking yourself these four questions:

1. Does your loved one not know how to solve the problem?
2. Is emotion interfering with her ability to start to solve the problem?
3. Does she lack confidence that she'll be able to identify the right solution or that she'll be able to implement the solution she chooses?
4. Are you having a problem with the way she's asking for help?

You might be able to guess the answers to questions 1 and 2 if you know this person very well and have a lot of past experience with such situations. Has your relative shown the ability to solve problems generally or this type of problem in particular? From what you know of her history and her body language right now, is fear, anger, or shame interfering with her ability to conceptualize and solve the problem?

As to question 3, your loved one might explicitly express a lack of confidence ("I know I have those three choices, but I always make the wrong choice!"), or, again, you might know from experience with her that she typically lacks such confidence.

And only you can say whether the way she's asking you for help is making you immediately want to refuse it. Some types of demands or pleas just push our hot buttons, and usually these are different for each individual—though there is one phrase that is offputting to just about everyone (see the box on this page).

If you are unsure of the answers to the four questions, your next step should be to do a little assessment with your loved one. She is asking for your help, and your help is contingent on having

> Does your loved one say "I need you to … "? In assertiveness training we teach clients never to request help using that phrase, because there is something about it that invariably makes everyone want to say no automatically.

more information. You'll recognize elements of the five-step response from Chapter 4 in the following exploration method:

1. *"What exactly is the problem? What needs to happen?"*

What you can do: If she cannot describe the problem or what outcome she wants, work with her to get a clear problem definition. As you go, gently work on solutions with her. Teach her problem solving (see the box on page 138), help her figure out the steps for her specific problems, and then get her to agree to try it. Don't forget to validate, validate, validate (see Chapter 3) at every step how difficult this is for her.

2. *"Are you afraid you can't get what you need to happen . . . too angry at that person to be effective . . . embarrassed that you need to do this?"*

What you can do: If this is the problem, have your relative check the facts of the situation. Often, emotion interferes with action because we are treating the emotions as fact. For example, if your loved one is afraid to talk to your partner about helping her fix something in her home, she should look at the facts. Can your partner actually do what she wants him to do? Is he likely to cause her physical or emotional harm if she asks? (If the answer really is yes, she shouldn't ask.) Is Paul really going to die of embarrassment at the bank? Help your loved one see that her emotions are just emotions and that she can solve the problem in spite of them, by saying something like: "I know you're afraid you're going to die of embarrassment, but no one ever really did. You can go to the bank even while you're embarrassed." "I know you're afraid he will say no. Here's the deal: you can ask him even if you're afraid."

3. *"Do you believe you're capable of solving the problem?"*

What you can do: This one is difficult. That lack of confidence is probably due to a long history of failing when trying to solve problems. Your telling your loved one that you have faith in her may be a little helpful but not sufficient. In reality, only the repetition of solving problems with success will breed confidence. Remember also that if you give in and solve the problem for her, you are undermining her confidence in the long run. If the problem is something like going to a bank or calling someone, you might offer to be with her but tell her that she is going to do all the talking. If the problem is at work or somewhere that you cannot be, you could offer to role-play the situation with her. Then make the role play as realistic as possible. In other words, have her tell you how the other person may respond. DBT therapists often role-play difficult situations with each other. Recently, I needed to have a difficult conversation with my supervisor. She is known for responding in ways that make me anxious. I was worried that I wouldn't be able to say what was needed, so a friend of mine (who knows my supervisor and how she is likely to react) role-played the situation with me. The act of having to think through my supervisor's responses made me more confident going into the conversation than I would have been without the practice.

4. *"Am I having a problem with the way I'm being asked to help? Do I immediately feel like saying no? Knowing the answers to questions 1–3, would I feel like helping was appropriate if I were asked differently?"*

What you can do: If you've determined that your loved one honestly doesn't know how to solve the problem, that emotions may be interfering with her objective analysis of the facts, and/or that her momentum is being halted by lack of confidence, what's stopping you from wanting to help her in a way that will encourage her to learn to handle these things on her own in the future? If your natural compassion for this person you care so much about is absent in this situation, it's probably because you've been told that you MUST help and you resent it, as most people would. When this happens, it's important to ask yourself if your knee-jerk response—saying no—is more about the fact that this is a problem that your loved one can solve on his own or more about the way that he's asking you to help. In other words, if the problem should be solved by your loved one, don't spend a lot of time on how he is approaching you for help. Spend time on how to solve the problem. However, if the problem is something that you are willing to assist with (a problem that anyone would need help solving) and the interpersonal style is what is making you want to say no, then ask your loved one to reframe how he is talking to you. This is very tricky and will almost always cause increased emotions in your loved one. If those increased emotions raise emotions in you too, go back to the methods for regulating your own emotion in Chapter 4.

Next, try the set of interpersonal skills that we teach in DBT for asking someone for what you want. Ultimately, it would be effective for your loved one to learn the skills, but if *you* use them to address his interpersonal style, you may find it works. The skills can be remembered with the acronym DEAR:

> **D:** Describe the situation. Just state the facts.
> **E:** Express your feelings and opinions about the situation.
> **A:** Assert your wishes. Ask your loved one for what you want.
> **R:** Reinforce/reward your loved one ahead of time for giving you what you want.

How would this look when talking to your loved one? You may need two DEARs, one to ask him to change how he is talking to you and one to say no to the request:

- *To say no to a request for help*

    D: Paul, you asked me to go to the bank to straighten out your account.

    E: I am not comfortable dealing with your money, and I think this is something you could do on your own.

    A: I am not going to the bank for you, but

    R: I will help you figure out exactly what you need to say if you will sit down with me and help me understand the situation.

- *To talk to someone about how he talks to you*

    D: Sarah: You are saying you want my help.

    E: When you tell me what to do with such a loud voice, it makes me not want to do it, even when I know helping you would be effective.

    A: Will you ask me again in a calmer, less judgmental voice?

    R: If you will do so, I will help you with your problem.

Because the relationship with your loved one is important to you, remember to be validating. You do know it's hard to ask people who are in power for help and that all of us have situations where we don't have confidence. If you need to get a compassion boost before initiating a conversation like this, see the suggestions in Chapter 4.

I once had a client who had a job but was on the verge of losing it because of cursing out her supervisor and finally having a cutting event that left blood in her office. When she came to see me, she was adamant that I intervene by telling her supervisor that he could not fire her. Of course I couldn't do that. I began to try to work with her on how she might appeal to her workplace. She did not believe she was capable and became more and more upset even though I was expressing belief in her and trying to help her find a solution. Finally, she slammed her palm down on my desk (so hard that several coworkers of mine came barging through the door to make sure I wasn't being assaulted) and yelled, "Dammit, you need to fix my life and fix it now!" She had all of the faith in the world in me and none in herself. This made her aggressive in trying to get me to help her. What I needed to do was to validate her enough to get her emotions down ("You are afraid of losing this job. You don't think you can do anything about it. Of course you want someone to help you"). Then I could work on solving the problems ("Look, you know, don't you, that it would not be effective for me to call your boss. It will just piss him off more. Let's figure out what you can do.").

As I got to know my client better, I found out that she had once lived with a family friend. That friend had asked her to leave because she felt that my client took advantage of her. My client couldn't understand what she had done. In her mind, she had been kind to this person, which I am sure she had. However, she had gotten her friend embroiled in a legal battle on my client's behalf, and the friend could not tolerate the emotionality that arose whenever there was anything to do regarding the legal situation. My client would talk badly about mutual friends and insist that her friend agree. She was relentless in her demands that her friend "take her side" and berated the friend when she did not. As part of our treatment, we worked on reestablishing a relationship with the friend. However, to do so, my client had to learn not to talk badly about their mutual friends to her and also had to learn how to act in a way that would make her friend want to help her. So, ultimately she had to learn how to solve problems on her own and how to deal with others in a way that made them want to help her when she needed help.

Reinforce Problem-Solving Efforts

I've given you a number of ideas for helping your loved one develop problem-solving skills if a lack of those skills is the main problem. I've also given you a way to try to improve communications between you if you know that there are times when a request for help is perfectly legitimate and yet you find yourself angry, defensive, and resistant just because of the way you're being spoken to. But if a big issue for your loved one is lack of confidence, it will also be important—again, only as long as you can do so sincerely and respectfully, without a hint of patronizing—to reinforce whatever attempts he makes to problem-solve. This doesn't mean you should ignore failures. On the contrary, if your 18-year-old son tried to take care of his own bank business and the bank refused to help him, you should do what you can to review what went wrong and what could be done differently. Naturally, you will start with validating the emotions your son is probably having about the outcome.

Just as important is that you don't validate the invalid: the poor decision or an ineffective action, like walking out on the bank manager while he was trying to talk with your son. It can be a fine line to tread, but just like with kids learning to accept that not everyone can be the best at everything, it's important to find a way to reinforce the effort and whatever went well while being honest (and nonblaming) about what didn't go well. The point is that many people with BPD already feel incompetent and ashamed of their perceived incompetence, and countering that learned self-image while validating the emotions they are feeling opens a door to learning problem-solving skills that usually stays closed when confidence is missing.

Encourage Emotional Regulation

If you know that your loved one is having trouble conceptualizing the problem and coming up with good solutions to test out because emotion always commandeers her brain, pay particular attention to the emotional regulation suggestions in Chapters 4 and 5. Having a "clear head" is a prerequisite for problem solving.

It's important for your loved one to try to learn to solve problems, not just to improve daily life and achieve long-term goals but also to prevent the emotional fallout of continued "failures" from growing. Chapter 8 describes "apparent competence," a borderline behavior in which some people effectively evade the whole issue of problem solving by acting as if everything is fine and they can handle whatever they are facing when, in actuality, they cannot.

"Things Are Awful ... but Don't Worry; I'm Handling It"

Katie's fiancé, Matt, looks totally capable of solving life's problems. To most of the people who know him, he's like any other adult in that way: He's made complicated travel plans for their sailing club. He's negotiated politically sensitive conflicts at the office. He can maneuver his SUV through the ice storms his area has every winter with skill. But Katie often sees another Matt, the one who calls her in a panic because he's been tasked with making a restaurant reservation for a work dinner and insists he can't do it. Katie is bewildered. She's seen him do it before. As a matter of fact, just a few weeks ago she met him for dinner at a new restaurant, where he had made a reservation in his name. Now, when he demands that she help him even though she's in the middle of what she considers a *real* work crisis, she first tries to joke him out of it: "Very funny, Matt. Sure, I'll help you. Reach into your pocket and pull out that little thing with the keys that we call a 'cell phone' and call Loretto's, your favorite, and ask for a table for 12 at 7:00." Instead of an appreciative laugh, however, she gets first dead silence and then a flat-toned "Oh. Yes. I can do that." Then Matt hangs up. Katie still feels a little confused but goes back to solving her own problems. When she gets home, Matt is waiting for her, and he looks pale and tells her in a shaky voice that he just couldn't make the dinner plans and he's going to lose his job unless she helps him.

Matt has BPD. Sometimes Katie and others who know him particularly well see him behave in the ways just described. When he begs for help with something they are convinced he can do on his own, he is engaging in active-passivity, described in Chapter 7. When he says in a matter-of-fact way, and believes, that he can handle a certain task and then demonstrates that he can't, he's engaging in what we call *apparent competence*. Apparent competence takes a number of different forms, but essentially it describes a pattern in which the person looks totally capable of solving the problems life presents but really is not.

Obviously this behavior can be problematic for those who love this person in a number of ways. Maybe you count on your loved one to handle certain tasks, only to find out they haven't been done. Maybe you end up in arguments because you assumed your sister or cousin could do something that she was sure she couldn't do. Do you ever find yourself feeling sure that you've seen the person with BPD do something before and now find she cannot do it? Do you ever feel like your experience of what is reality is dramatically different from her experience of reality? Does your loved one ever tell you that everything is okay when, in fact, some area of her life is falling apart?

In Chapter 1 we talked about all the ways that BPD can make you feel so lost in your relationship. Apparent competence can be a huge factor in making you feel adrift. You thought you knew your loved one's capabilities and now wonder if you were imagining things. Who is this person who operates with such ease in college classes but then can't seem to function as an adult within his family? How is it that your loved one has just threatened to do something drastic out of despair over a failing relationship when just an hour ago she was telling you with a smile all about how she would talk to her friend about their argument, apologize for her part in it, and make sensible changes in the way she deals with this person who's so important to her?

Like Matt, Linda repeatedly shows an ability to deal with very intricate and important interpersonal issues at work. She manages a team of people, and they work very well with her. However, when she is at home, she is anxious and depressed and she can't seem to ask her husband to do the most mundane household chores. Her resentment is building and building because he won't do things like take out the trash, make sure the cat is fed, or water the lawn. What Linda could handle easily at work seems to be an impossibility at home.

Jordan is sitting in her mother's kitchen, telling her about having seen her boyfriend kissing another girl in between classes and then the two of them spotting Jordan and laughing right in her face. She describes the scene in a monotone, without facial expression or inflection, as if she were reading a boring speech written by someone in the 1600s. She really doesn't appear to be impacted by what she is telling her mother even though her words say otherwise. So her mother's response is minimal and matches her daughter's tone of voice more than the contents of the story she is telling. Later that day, Jordan's mother finds out from her other daughter that Jordan was in fact devastated. After gulping a bottle of wine while on the phone with her sister, Jordan calls her mother and berates her for being as cruel as her cheating boyfriend and "that tramp." Jordan believes she clearly communicated her shock, heartbreak, and humiliation. Jordan's mother can't figure out how Jordan could have seemed so calm if she had felt that bad and why her daughter wouldn't have more accurately communicated how catastrophic the incident was for her.

Kali's aunt is relieved to see that she seems to be handling life well these days. At the Fourth of July barbecue she seems relaxed and not defensive as she used to be. Her mood seems light. She smiles; she laughs; she teases her like she used to but never with an edge of meanness. She doesn't seem at all depressed. Then, 4 hours after leaving her home, Kali calls and says that she is horribly depressed and that her aunt's not realizing how depressed she is has made her feel worse. Kali feels let down by her lack of responsiveness, and now her aunt feels confused and let down herself that she did not see what her niece says was a glaring reality.

Apparent competence can manifest itself in a lot of different ways, and recognizing them all can help you figure out the best way to respond. Several things may happen in apparent competence. For one, there may be a problem of generalization. That is, you may be baffled by the fact that your loved one can engage in some behaviors in one context but not in others. For another, you may unwittingly complicate matters by treating your loved one like she has capabilities she doesn't have. Third, your loved one may be "masking emotions," which can lead you to think things are okay when your loved one is actually ready to explode. Finally, it may be that your loved one brightens up when she is in your presence and then crashes when the interaction with you is over. Let's look at each of these more closely.

$\mathcal{C}$an Your Loved One Generalize the Ability to Do Something?

Animals, including all human beings, learn behaviors in one context; this is called *situation-specific learning*. In her very helpful book on shaping behavior (*Don't Shoot the Dog!*), Karen Pryor, a dolphin trainer, explains that dolphins can't take a trick from one tank to another. So, a dolphin that is beautifully trained in one Sea World must be retrained when later moved to another. Behaviors simply don't move from one context (environment) to another. A young child may learn to be quiet in school but then have to be taught to do the same thing at religious services. To the child the context that demands quiet is the classroom, which is not the same as the place of worship. Eventually the child may be able to identify two different settings as having the same operative context because of some important feature they share. For example, a slightly older child may be able to figure out that quiet is required in a museum where a curator is lecturing because other people are being quiet and because someone is speaking to a group whose members are actively listening, or at a concert because people are being quiet and loud talking would prevent them from hearing the music. A still older child may figure out that being quiet is a way of showing respect at a somber occasion such as a funeral.

In addition to the difficulty that all animals have with generalizing behavior from one environmental context to the other, people with BPD have emotional and cognitive dysregulation, which further compound problems with generalization. All human beings have to make mental associations in order to generalize. However, high emotional arousal makes generalization almost impossible for people with BPD. Researchers have done many studies on how people learn new behaviors. They have found that people who learn behaviors in one place will not necessarily be able to repeat them somewhere else. People who have been suicidal or who are currently depressed have less ability to translate behavior from context to context. High emotional arousal decreases the chance that people can perform tasks. If your loved one is more regulated at home than at work, she may look more capable at home. Your loved one's mood state affects her ability to engage in behaviors in different places. If she is more anxious and depressed at home, behavioral control and expression will be more difficult at home.

The problem is that people surrounding someone with BPD get exasperated by the fact that certain behaviors are evident in some contexts but not others. It's easy to look at your loved one and say, "Jim can have a disagreement with his father and calm down, but he disagrees with me and things get really out of control." Then family members get judgmental: "He doesn't want to control himself." Wanting, however, may not enter into it at all. It could be that the situation is different or that the mood is different. It could also be that the reinforcers are different.

People with BPD seem to have more trouble generalizing behaviors than others largely because, as with so many of their other problems, emotions interfere with learning. High emotional arousal can not only inhibit the use of an already learned behavior but also block further learning about the appropriate use of that behavior. I am a person who can be pretty interpersonally skillful. I know all of the assertiveness skills required to get people to do things for me. I really struggle to get airlines to do things for me, however, because I have a hard time using my interpersonal skills with airline agents. Usually I need these skills when flights are canceled or something is happening to keep me from getting where I am going. My frustration and other emotions are very high at those times. It's not that I don't know the words; I just can't get them out because of my arousal. As long as I can't change the arousal, I can't apply my interpersonal skills fully; nor can I learn a new way to deal effectively with airline employees. All I can do to solve this problem is to start making my requests when I am not in a state of high emotion.

> If your loved one seems unable to do something in one context that she can do in another, it's not that she isn't trying hard enough; it's that the behaviors literally are not in her repertoire of behaviors for that specific environment.

Because people with BPD can become so overwhelmed by emotion, a simple task can be harder for them in a context that many people would view as less, not more, challenging. This is why others think that the person with BPD ought to be able to complete the tasks and don't believe their loved one when they say it is impossible. Take Linda as an example. Many people would feel too intimidated by business colleagues, who are judging their worth at work, to give orders and handle office politics, whereas their trust in their loved ones makes it easy for them to insist that a spouse do a fair share of chores. But Linda, afraid of abandonment, like many people with BPD, feels more threatened by the possible disapproval of her husband than of her associates at the office.

Moods Become a Context

What compounds the problem for people with BPD is that they not only don't have a great ability to generalize behavior across contexts, but they also are mood dependent. So, the abilities that your loved one has in one context (let's say in dealing with her relationship with you) change depending on her mood state.

Let's say yesterday you were having lunch with Tasha, who was in a very peaceful emotional place. She said she had been sleeping well and felt like she was making progress in her life. Tasha asked your opinion on whether she should go out with a man she met on the Internet. You told her you thought she should talk with him on the phone and then meet for lunch. She accepted your opinion and said it was good advice even though it was not what she really wanted to hear—she said she wished you had told her that you think the guy sounds great and she should "go for it."

Today Tasha calls you and is very emotionally aroused. Her voice is loud, and her speech is quick. She says she is so excited that she barely slept last night. Before she went to bed, she got an e-mail from the man she has been talking to on the Internet, asking her to go away with him for the weekend because he has a place at the beach. She asks you what you think, and you repeat what you said yesterday. She becomes enraged by your response and tells you that you don't really care about her and you want her to spend her life alone. Yesterday she could accept your opinion even if she didn't agree with it. Today she cannot. What is the difference? The difference is mood state. It could be that her emotions were well regulated yesterday and today she is very excited about seeing the guy. She did not sleep, which makes all of us more sensitive to emotion. However, her ability to process the feedback that you give her is entirely dependent on her mood state. The advice didn't change, but the situation did and her emotions did.

Of course we all have problems with generalization, and we can have problems with our emotions and mood interfering with our behavior. Have you ever tried to quit smoking? If so, I'll bet there were some places where not smoking was easy for you, maybe because it was a place where smoking wasn't allowed or because it was a place where you didn't smoke when you were a smoker. Other places were more difficult, but you had your plan of alternative behaviors (twist an arm band, suck on a Lifesaver) that worked for you. Then you would go to your friend's home. This friend is a smoker, and you used to sit on her back porch and smoke cigarettes. At that moment everything that you knew worked kind of went out the window. You still had the same arm band and Lifesavers in your purse, and you were just as committed to not smoking, but it just didn't happen. You didn't generalize behaviors from one environment to the next.

Now, thinking about the effect of your mood on not smoking, let's say you had a really bad day and were angry and disgusted. Then you went to your friend's house and your friend was sitting on her back porch smoking. You might just light up a cigarette without even thinking about it. Or you might say "to heck with it" and then light up a cigarette. If she wasn't smoking, though, and didn't have cigarettes, you might not smoke either. Your behavior depends on context (the environment, the availability) *and your mood.*

Knowing that this connection is even stronger for those with BPD should give you a clue about what could be going on when your loved one's apparent competence gives way to demonstrated incompetence. In the case of Matt, it might not be that he was invalidating himself regard-

---

When you're confused and exasperated by your loved one's "sudden" inability to do something you've seen him do before, ask yourself:

- Have you *ever* seen him demonstrate this ability in this particular context? If not, it may be because he hasn't generalized this behavior.
- Does this context tap into an emotional vulnerability you're aware of in your relative?
- Do you know what your loved one's mood is right now (anxious? depressed? overexcited? irritated? etc.)?

ing his ability to apply social skills in the business setting. It could have been that his mood was anxious that day for completely unconnected reasons. Those who don't have BPD can often regulate their emotions so that those emotions don't affect something unrelated. You might be able to set aside your anxiety over a medical test so that it wouldn't hamper your ability to pick a restaurant, make the reservation, and not worry excessively about your choice. But Matt might not have been able to do this. Katie might not have known what her fiancé's mood was when he called her, but knowing that mood could have played a big role might have helped her react differently.

$\mathcal{A}$re You Making Assumptions That Lead to Invalidation?

A second possibility to consider when your loved one's ability to perform certain tasks seems to come and go is whether you're making assumptions you shouldn't make. Are you sure your loved one really has the capability you're attributing to her? Sometimes we *think* people are more capable than they are. Sometimes that's because we have seen the behavior before and just expect a person to repeat it. For example, Justine is trying to quit cutting herself. For Justine, an argument with you is a cue (something that usually starts the ball rolling in such a way that Justine ends up self-harming). You are in control of Justine's money. You don't want to be, but it seemed the effective thing to do since she always overspent and then came to you for help. Several times, after a disagreement about how to distribute Justine's money, she has had cutting episodes. A few weeks ago Justine came to you and said that she wanted money to put down on a car. You went through the budget with her and explained that she did not have the financial stability to make a car payment. Justine was disappointed but handled her emotional distress.

Then, a few days later, she comes to you for money for a new pair of boots. Because you already had the discussion about the car, you just respond, "Justine, you know you can't afford it. I'm not writing a check." Because she tolerated that "bad" news about the car so well, you think she can tolerate being told no about the boots. But she doesn't; she becomes very upset and ends up cutting herself. What happened? Probably several things. You assumed that because Justine could tolerate disappointment once, in what you considered to be a more disappointing circumstance, she could tolerate it again.

But just because Justine could engage in emotion-moderating behavior on one occasion doesn't mean she can repeat the behavior. It could be that Justine has had several disappointments during the day. Maybe she didn't sleep. There are an infinite number of factors that could make her more vulnerable to being denied the boots. Some of them have to do with difficulty generalizing, as just discussed.

It's not that you need to be able to determine exactly how far and how deeply your loved one's competence in a certain area extends. It's that you should always be willing to consider the possibility that *apparent* competence is not always *actual* competence, and therefore whenever your loved one appears not to be able to do something you thought she could do, *she probably really cannot do it, at least not there and then.*

> *Apparent competence often means that the environment treats your loved one as someone who is more skillful than he or she is.*

Do not assume that your loved one is more capable than he is!

If you think that your loved one is more capable that she thinks she is (or than she really is), you will inadvertently invalidate her. You will communicate to her that she could have done whatever the behavior was "if you had really wanted to"—that she wasn't trying hard enough or that she was "manipulating" or "playing games." In the example with Justine, it would be easy for the

---

If you think your loved one should be able to do something he's done before, ask yourself:

- How do I know he has the skill to do this in virtually every situation?
- Am I assuming he's playing games to get me to do something he could do for himself?

Drawing a hard-line conclusion that you *know* your loved one can do what's required, and therefore judging him manipulative when he says he can't, is a sure sign that you're imposing potentially faulty assumptions that invalidate.

family member to think that because Justine cut herself after the tennis shoe incident she was "playing games" to get her family member to buy new shoes for her or change her mind about allowing her to purchase them. If you think about what we have already discussed (generalization and mood dependency), it is probably that Justine really couldn't tolerate the disappointment about the shoes and/or her lack of sleep and other disappointments set her up to be unable to deal with another disappointment. The problem here, though, was that Justine's family member assumed that because she could tolerate disappointment on one day about one issue, she could always tolerate disappointment.

*I*s Your Loved One Masking Emotion?

Apparent competence is often the end result of masking emotion. People mask emotions when they don't allow what they are experiencing emotionally to show on their faces or in their physical movements. One of the things that emotions do is to communicate our experience to others and thereby influence their behaviors. For example, you can usually tell that someone is angry at you from facial expressions (frowning, brows furrowed), nonverbal behaviors (arms crossed, hands clenched), and verbal expression (rapid speech, loud voice, and words). People with BPD often automatically inhibit the nonverbal behaviors associated with negative emotions. They may do this for several reasons:

1. As children, they may have learned that demonstrating (or even having) negative emotion is inappropriate.
2. Over time, their demonstration of negative emotion has been punished by the environment, sometimes because the emotional behavior has been over the top and out of control but sometimes just because there was any emotional behavior.

As people with BPD repeatedly get into trouble because of their emotions, they develop a disconnect between their emotions and the expression of them. They begin to shut down (we will talk about this in a later chapter), but they also begin to inhibit the natural expression of their emotions, or at least try to. The result is sometimes an incongruence between what the person with BPD is experiencing emotionally and how it is expressed outwardly. In masking, emotions are still there; they just aren't allowed to have their natural expression. So people with BPD may be really angry but laugh or may be really sad but tell you that they are all right in a voice that sounds all right, even though they aren't fine at all.

> Masking is not an effort at "manipulation" or an attempt to control other people. It's an adaptive response to a history of problematic experiences with out-of-control emotions.

Have you ever had your loved one tell you that this was the worst day of her life? She tells you the story of what has happened, and it does sound really horrendous, but she tells you this while flipping through a magazine and with an expression on her face that doesn't communicate "worst day of my life." She is not teary, her voice isn't thready, her facial muscles do not seem tight. You have known your loved one to have really bad days and totally fall apart, so since she does not *look* to you like she is falling apart, you don't respond to her like this is the worst day of her life. Your response is somewhat in keeping with her reading the magazine. You may say some supportive things, but you are not jumping in there and saying "This is TERRIBLE. What are we going to do?" as you would if someone else you know said the same thing. The problem with masking and your responding to your loved one as if she is more competent than she feels right now is that it may actually be one of the worst days of her life. She may, in fact, feel out of control and suicidal and is not accurately expressing this to you. It is important to know that your loved one may believe that describing what she feels as opposed to showing you what she feels is sufficient to demonstrate the level of her emotion. She may not understand that people will automatically respond to nonver-

---

If your loved one is describing a horrible experience but without emotional expression, ask yourself:

- How would you (or anyone else) feel in this situation? If your answer is "horrible," then trust the words, not the expression.
- Describe the difference between what you are seeing and what you are hearing to your loved one and ask her which is correct.

bal expressions of emotion over verbal expressions of emotion. If your response is tempered or lukewarm, she may then become very angry at you or hopeless that even you don't understand how bad things truly are for her.

7s Your Loved One Gaining Competence from Your Support?

Finally, sometimes people with BPD can seem more competent than they really are when they are in the room with someone who is nurturing and supportive. Therapists see this all the time: The person with BPD seems to be doing well in a therapy session but then calls later in the day, saying that her life is so desperate that she is going to kill herself. Even therapists are confused by this shift: Why didn't the client didn't tell the therapist this? The answer is that the issue was not present when the client was in the room with the therapist. When the external cues of the nurturing environment are gone, the distressing emotions return. The client really didn't feel suicidal while she was with the therapist, but those thoughts and feelings returned when the session was over.

> Remember, people with BPD are largely relational people.

Those with BPD are "people who need people" as the song goes. They don't like to be alone and function better when they are in supportive, caring relationships. Often, there is a dearth of caring relationships in the lives of people with BPD, so if your loved one has one of the caring relationships with you, chances are her emotions will be better regulated at times just because she is with you or talking to you. Then, when she is alone again, loneliness crashes in on her, all of the despairing, hopeless emotions return, and the dysregulation returns. Neither of you is doing anything wrong. It is just that your nurturing presence makes your loved one feel better.

What You Can Do in the Face of Apparent Competence

Now you've seen the various features of apparent competence separately, but it's important to know that they can occur together. Take the example of Leo. Leo often looks as if he is more competent in some contexts than he really is. He works as a corporate sales manager and is well liked by his coworkers, who find him funny and charming. They don't know that going to work causes Leo tremendous anxiety. When he gets anxious, he misses meetings with his accounts and falsifies his reports. Leo is worried that at any minute his supervisor is going to find out that he has been missing meetings with clients. Because he appears to be doing well, Leo's supervisor increases the size of his sales territory. This, of course, increases his anxiety, and now his worry that he is going to lose his job is out of control. You have some idea about what is happening, but he assures you that he has everything under control. At home, Leo is very good at getting projects done even when they make him anxious, so you have no reason to believe that he cannot manage his anxiety. Plus, he is saying all is well. And, when you and he are at home together, he looks calm and tells you he believes he can make it. Then he comes home one day and tells you he's sure he's going to lose his job—but he has a plan. Leo's confidence seems high and he actually encourages you. You have had a pretty bad day yourself, so you are just relieved that he has everything under control. Then, the next week, he actually does lose his job and is devastated. You also are devastated, because of the implications of his job loss but also because you believed he had everything under control. He becomes suicidal when you confront him because he cannot believe that you couldn't see that he really was worried and anxious about his job. Of course, now you are feeling emotionally out of control because Leo doesn't have a job and because you are no longer sure how to communicate with Leo.

The most important thing to do with apparent competence is to remember the behavioral patterns. Just being aware that your loved one may not be feeling on the inside what she is showing on the outside will lead you to ask questions like the ones in the boxes earlier in this chapter and to be cautious about expecting behaviors that your loved one may not be capable of using. Do not get judgmental or think that your loved one is "pretending." Apparent competence is not a pretend state. It happens when the environment is affecting the behavior of your loved one. Either (1) being with you in a supportive caring environment lessens your loved one's emotional response to his problems; (2) your loved one, for a number of reasons, has emotions and nonverbal behaviors that are not congruent in certain circumstance; or (3) your loved one's behaviors have not generalized from context to context. Your loved one is not trying to "put one over" on you but is engaging in behaviors that have developed over time.

Use the Five-Step Response

You can also use the five-step response described in Chapter 4. This might work particularly well with situations like the one involving Tasha:

1. *Regulate your own emotion.* You made the assumption that Tasha could hear advice she didn't want to hear no matter what the context, so naturally you might feel frustrated or angry when she blows up at you for giving the same advice she accepted yesterday. Remember that her behavior is mood dependent. If you notice her shift in mood between yesterday and today, you'll be able to remind yourself that this means the context is different and so might her response be.

2. *Validate.* When Tasha explodes, tell her you understand this isn't the advice she wanted to hear and it must feel terrible to hope you've found someone and then be advised to take it slow in pursuing him.

3. *Ask/assess.* Ask her what her own concerns are: Why is she asking your opinion again? Could it be that she has her own doubts? What could she do to figure out the wise move?

4. *Brainstorm/troubleshoot.* If she does want your opinion because she's really not sure what to do, help her list her options for learning more about this man as well as options for getting together with him while ensuring her own safety. Troubleshoot the best options.

5. *Get information on your role (if any) and what you can plan on hearing about the outcome.* Does Tasha want to check in with you while she's pursuing the course of action she's chosen and get your feedback along the way? Do you want her to get in touch after she meets the man to let you know she's okay and tell you how it went?

Know Your Loved One's Limitations, but Don't Fragilize

Shifting into this five-step response can defuse misunderstandings fueled by apparent competence. But in many cases you also have to make sure you really understand what it is that your loved one is feeling—since masking emotion is so often behind displays of apparent competence—and what your loved one is capable of doing. This means not treating your loved one like he is fragile and, at the same time, not having unrealistic expectations of his behavior. If you are thinking that your loved one's behavior is not generalizing from situation to situation and if you are aware that she may not be accurately communicating her vulnerabilities to you, the tendency is for you to try to intervene for your loved one and do things for her. Doing so, of course, reinforces your loved one's belief that she cannot do things for herself. It also does not allow your loved one to practice behaviors in new environments, thus increasing generalization.

What do you do?

1. *Don't assume competence.* This doesn't mean don't give disappointing news, etc. Don't think that because you have seen a behavior before, it means that it is going to come out again. Don't believe that your loved one can do things because his peers can do them.

2. *Balance intervening with coaching.* It is easy to think that because behaviors don't generalize and because moods and emotions make a greater impact on people with BPD than people without BPD, we should intervene on their behalf. In fact, it often seems like it would just be easier on us all if we did whatever it is for our loved one. However, this sends the message that the person is fragile and cannot do things on his own. Make sure the person has the requisite behaviors and can use them in this situation before jumping to conclusions about why your loved one seems unable to do something you thought he could do. In the case of Justine and the boots, take the time to make sure she is tolerating the news and don't just plunge in as if she can take the bad news well.

3. *Remember the effect of mood and emotion on generalization*: If you are quitting smoking, you may quit visiting your friend or quit sitting on her back porch. You may not go to her house when you have had a really bad day. Part of your job as a family member is to be aware of generalization problems so that you are not disappointed if your loved one does not generalize a behavior. This will help you keep your arousal down and will keep you from having pejorative thoughts about your loved one. It is easier on us all if we are not thinking that we are being "manipulated" or "played."

If you are concerned that your loved one is apparently competent because he is masking emotions, say things like, "You really don't look hor-

ribly upset about this. Are you not terribly upset, or are you dying inside and not telling me?" You may also ask your loved one to tell you what she is feeling inside her body.

Now you can respond in an effective manner to the actual emotion and not to your loved one's presentation of the emotion. The important thing to remember about apparent competence is the word *appear*. There are situations where your loved one will actually *be* competent. We all have them, and some of what we do for our loved ones is find the places where they are competent and build them up. But people around those with BPD often treat them as if they are competent in context when they are not. This adds to their sense of not being understood or being so pathological that they cannot be understood and will increase their emotional dysregulation in the moment. Emotional dysregulation can lead to a pattern of unrelenting crisis, as described in the next chapter.

"Why Do Terrible Things Keep Happening to Me?"

You just don't understand Kristy. She never seems to get her life in order. She moves from crisis to crisis to crisis. She finally gets the job at the museum that she's always wanted but then bounces a check after going on a shopping spree for clothes "with just the right artistic look." When the store calls her at work and gets her boss, she's so mortified that she stays home for 3 days without calling in. When she gets fired, she drinks two bottles of wine and leaves a threatening voice mail for her ex-supervisor, who calls the police. When the police show up at her door, she explains how upset she was and that it was a one-time event that will never happen again. She seems so calm and rational that the police are reassured. As soon as they leave, Kristy goes into the bathroom and starts cutting her thighs. She calls you and says she wants to die. You call 911, and she is admitted to the hospital. You fear it's only a matter of time once she's released before the cycle begins again.

You and Kristy are in what we call *unrelenting crisis*. Maybe you've begun to think that Kristy actually enjoys having her life in an uproar. It seems as if there's no gap between times when she calls and asks you to fix the latest mess and times when you see a crisis build and build like a thunderstorm until the tension is too much and Kristy ends up in a suicidal state, landing again in the psychiatric hospital.

Unrelenting crisis is exhausting for both of you. It leaves Kristy more and more desperate, more and more convinced that she can't do anything right and that you and everyone else who cares about her will abandon her any minute. It leaves you feeling helpless, frustrated, probably alternately furious and terrified. You may be reaching a point where you dread seeing Kristy, hearing from her, even learning the latest news about her life from a distance.

If you've reached that point, the first thing I need to tell you is that *some of the crises are not of your loved one's creation.* People with BPD often have catastrophic physical problems. There is a constellation of problems called the *depressive five*—temporomandibular joint disorder (TMJ), migraines, fibromyalgia, irritable bowel syndrome (IBS), and interstitial cystitis—that is very common among those with BPD, along with myasthenia gravis and rheumatoid arthritis. Physical pain and discomfort make all of us more vulnerable to emotion, and as you can imagine, for someone who is highly emotionally vulnerable these physiological conditions just make things worse, making additional crises even more likely. Physical conditions like these also may cause your loved one financial stress, job stress, and relationship stress, leading to crisis from those secondary problems.

Unfortunately, those with BPD seem to be acutely sensitive to physical discomfort and react emotionally to it, which makes them talk about their conditions all the time. Because of apparent competence, people with BPD can describe their physical and emotional pain without showing how bad they feel. This makes people question its authenticity and the person's motivation for talking about it. Naturally, this can increase tensions between others and the person who has BPD plus a physical problem like one of the depressive five. And it sometimes leads observers to suspect that the physical problems are either nonexistent or greatly exaggerated. If you've fallen prey to that suspicion, rest assured that fibromyalgia, rheumatoid arthritis, irritable bowel syndrome, and myasthenia gravis are considered "true" diagnoses. And your loved one is unlikely to be overstating his pain, physical or emotional.

Similarly, people with BPD often have other psychiatric problems, such as depression, anxiety, and posttraumatic stress disorder. It's probably not hard to imagine that these psychiatric problems impose more stress on your loved one because they make it harder to function in everyday life. Any additional stress is going to compound the likelihood of crises occurring, through no fault of your loved one's own.

Kristy, for example, suffers from debilitating migraines. Jimmy, your younger brother, also has been burdened with pressures aside from BPD. Jimmy has had a difficult time in life. He struggled academically in high school. He was always in trouble and seemed to hang out with the "wrong" crowd. There was a lot of conflict at home with your parents, and Jimmy would disappear for days after a fight with them. After graduating, Jimmy joined the military. When he returned from the war, he was diagnosed

> *The chances of crises occurring increases when a person who has BPD is struggling with physical problems and/or other psychiatric conditions as well.*

with posttraumatic stress disorder and BPD and discharged. Jimmy has flashbacks if there are loud noises but can only get a job at a construction company. If there is any kind of crash at the construction site, Jimmy has flashbacks to the point of having to leave work. Then, instead of going someplace to get help for his problems (he refuses treatment), Jimmy goes to a bar to make the pain go away. Inevitably he gets into fights at the bar, and he has spent a couple of nights in jail. The local police have said that he will be charged if he gets into another fight. You are watching this situation build and build and know that an arrest is inevitable. When you try to talk with Jimmy, he explodes. There seems to be no way to keep Jimmy from the inevitable crash.

As with Jimmy, the crises of people with BPD often build over time. Because of their emotional vulnerability and reactivity, their initial emotional response to a problem is extreme. Then, before their emotions can drop to a more manageable level, something else happens to trigger another crisis. To some extent it's just that events in life ebb and flow—difficult events happen with regularity. If you're not emotionally vulnerable, you can usually roll with many of the challenges that life presents, or you can recover quickly enough to regain your emotional footing before the next tide comes in. People with BPD, as you now know, are more emotionally reactive and their emotions stick around a lot longer. If they are still reeling from one blow when another one comes at them, a larger crisis is likely to ensue. Also, if, like many people with BPD, they have not learned to solve problems adeptly (see Chapter 7), their response to one of the blows life tends to deliver may be inadequate, and the result is more crisis. Sometimes, because they don't have adequate interpersonal skills (see Chapter 7), the way those with BPD deal with the people who are either a part of the crisis or could help them solve the problem is not helpful, and their emotions increase even more. Usually, the person with BPD makes a series of decisions that don't solve the problem but make the problem worse.

First Dave's brother died of a heart attack. No one was expecting it. He seemed to be healthy. Dave's parents were devastated. Then, a few days after returning from the funeral, Dave found out that his company was closing and he was being laid off. Dave began drinking to help the pain and fear go away. When his wife yelled at him for drinking too much, he held a gun to his head and was taken to the hospital.

Laura loved purses. Lots of stores on the Internet knew she loved purses and sent her ads for "deals" on designer purses. She just couldn't help herself. She bought more than 20 designer purses, and her charge cards were maxed out. Then her car broke down and she had no money to fix it and she couldn't charge the repair costs. She didn't see any way out except for suicide.

Jill was having a hard time. The stress in her life was getting out of her control. Her boys were adolescents. They needed driving every-where. They were in sports and other extracurricular activities. Her hus-band had taken a job that required him to travel during most weeks. She already felt alone enough, then her best friend moved. She was completely overwhelmed by the stress and felt like she just needed a break. She got into her car and drove to the airport to fly away some-where. When she got to the parking lot, she was more overwhelmed and despondent. She pulled her medications out of her purse and swallowed them with a bottle of soda.

$\mathcal{A}$cting on Impulse: Cause or Effect?

In Chapter 1, I listed behavior as one of the five areas of dysregulation in BPD and impulsive behavior as one form that dysregulation takes. A common refrain among those who love someone with the disorder is "What were you *thinking*?" as if the person was just having a pleasant day and suddenly decided to do something crazy without thinking about what would follow in the future. In fact, though, people embroiled in unrelenting crisis are often *reacting* to what is *already happening*. They are in the midst of an overwhelming crisis right now, and a lot of impulsive behavior is pursued as a way to make the crisis end. Suicidal behaviors, self-harm, drinking, going to hospitals, running away—all of these so-called impulsive actions are intended to end the current crisis, whether it's Kristy's losing her job or Jimmy's experiencing combat flashbacks. What your loved one doesn't realize is that the behaviors applied to end the crises often cause crises of their own. All the person knows is that she has to do something—fast—to make the pain and turmoil cease.

Going to the hospital after harming herself really does interrupt the crisis for Kristy. Going to jail might actually end it for Jimmy. Emotions subside, the person gets a break from the people who may have been involved in the crisis, and social workers make helpful interventions. All of these consequences are good things for your loved one. Unfortunately, once Kristy is discharged from the hospital, she finds she now has a big financial burden from the hospital charges and missed work, and this financial burden becomes the beginning (or maybe the continuation if finances were a part of the prehospital crisis) of the next crisis.

You, of course, still want to know why your loved one couldn't foresee that a measure that solves one problem but creates another isn't the best choice. As I've described in earlier chapters, the answer is that your loved one has cognitive problems, such as having trouble paying attention when emotion is crowding out thoughts, and also lacks the skills of problem solving. The emotions that are fueling the crises are intense and feel out of control. As you'll see later in this chapter, this means that emotional regulation and problem solving can be good ways to exit the land of unrelenting crisis.

> The way out of unrelenting crisis is likely to be a combination of emotional regulation and use of problem-solving skills.

When impulsive actions are both the effect of a crisis and the cause of a crisis, however, it can be tough to figure out where you can step in and hope to disrupt the cycle. Imagine that your wife was at work one day and received an employee evaluation that was upsetting to her. She went back to her desk, wrote a resignation letter, and left her job. When you came home that night and she told you what she had done, you were upset with her. There was an argument. Your wife stormed out of the house, went to a bar, drank too much, and slept with another man. This caused more stress in your marriage, and your finances were stretched beyond capacity by the loss of her job. Your wife was overwhelmed with shame and regret and started diligently staying at home to find jobs. But soon she got bored, so instead of sticking to job searches online, she started browsing investment opportunities to make some quick money and spent most of your savings. When you got furious with her, there was another argument. During the argument, your wife went to the bathroom and took an overdose of pills. The ambulance was called, and she was taken to the hospital. You did not know that she had not signed up for COBRA insurance ("Because I was too mad at that place to deal with it"). Her hospitalization was therefore not covered, and now you owe $30,000 in medical costs. You don't have any hope that things are going to be better when your wife is discharged.

*W*hen Crisis Is Entrenched

You may know from personal experience that when a crisis situation is chronic, it can be particularly hard to extricate yourself. Some people stay mired in financial disaster from spending habits they can't seem to change because it would mean abandoning a familiar lifestyle. Some eat the same diet for years even though it causes them health problems, including emergencies at times. And some people tolerate miserable partnerships even when they are repeatedly abused physically or verbally.

Your daughter is married to a man who constantly berates her and tells her that she will never amount to anything. He only "allows" her to have a part-time job. She has no education, just a GED. Your daughter's husband requires that she stay at home when she is not working. Your daughter is very frightened about what would happen if she defied him. She believes (probably rightly) that she cannot leave her husband because she couldn't survive financially. She has looked at taking courses online to learn some skills, but she cannot afford it. She is becoming more and more depressed. You could give her the money to leave, but when you gave her the money to avoid filing for bankruptcy last year, you told her you were not giving her money again. Recently she has confided in you that she is pregnant. She believes that having a child will solve all of her problems. You know that the child is only going to create more problems, but your daughter is not hearing what you say. Watching your daughter is like watching a slow-motion train wreck. You can see the negative consequences coming.

*P*oor Judgment plus Poor Problem Solving

Most of the time, people with BPD do not intend to start the snowball of crisis behaviors that end up with catastrophic consequences. They engage in impulsive behaviors, and their problem-solving capabilities are negligible, so they make problematic decisions. The problems that arise are often a result of poor judgment compounded by poor problem solving.

Bella is a 50-year-old woman whose suicidal behavior is often fueled by financial and relationship stress. She has a job that pays her adequately, but she has no health insurance and no discernible retirement savings. She lives from paycheck to paycheck, largely because of her spending habits. She drinks a bottle of wine every night and smokes one to two packs of cigarettes a day. She spends any extra money she has going away for weekends at nice hotels and flying to New York City. Bella often has to borrow money from friends the week before she is paid. She recently received $25,000 in a divorce settlement. Instead of using the money to pay off her car or rent, she has decided to go on a cruise and have plastic surgery. She does not see that she would be better served paying bills and saving money for emergencies. She has asked her loved ones for their advice about the plastic surgery, but when they disagree with her plans, she ignores their input. Of course, she argues against their opinions and causes stress in her relationships. She is attached to the idea that she will feel better if she looks younger. She doesn't see that she is avoiding the emotions of the failed marriage. Several people have told her that they will no longer help her out when she needs help if she spends the money in ways they consider frivolous. Bella is not realistic in her assessment of her current financial situation or issues that could arise in the future. Her plan is to find another husband who will help her if she needs financial assistance.

I had a client once who went to the grocery store for food for her children and came home with a man who worked in the milk department. The client had many current stressors in her life. She lived on financial aid, she had a debilitating joint disease that caused her a lot of pain, and she was not equipped to care for her children, financially, emotionally, or physically. Her daughters lived with their father, and my client only had visitation for 2 weeks per year. During the visitation periods, my client was overwhelmed by the stress of caring for the girls. When she went to the store, she had never seen the man in the milk department before, but they began talking and she found out that he had just left his wife and had nowhere to stay. Within half an hour, she had taken him home and moved him in with her and her two visiting children. In 2 weeks, the client had lost visitation altogether because it turned out that the man was a sex offender and had attempted to molest her daughter. When the police came to her home to arrest the man and brought social services to take the children, my client became extremely upset and took off in her car. Because she was so emotional, she didn't drive well and hit another car. The driver of the car ended up in intensive care, and my client began to dwell on the problems that had fallen on her. She made a near lethal suicide attempt and ended up in the hospital. When she came to her session with me, it took me a long time to get my client to see that many of her behaviors had led to the problems that ensued.

Of course my client had no intention of losing her children, bringing a sex offender into her home, or becoming dysregulated to the point of a suicide attempt. Her behavior got out of control. She had behaved impulsively in meeting a man and immediately taking him home. When I found out, I talked with her about getting him out of the house, at least until her daughters left (I had no idea he was a sex offender). She left my office sure that she had the skills to tell him he had to leave, but then later reported that he "looked at me with his beautiful blue eyes" and she could not ask him to leave. She had intuitive thoughts that the man could be more interested in her daughter than he was in her, but she ignored them and focused on not being alone and enjoying her time with a new man.

The sequence of events resulted from a series of impulsive decisions and from ignoring the facts, with catastrophic consequences for my client and her daughters. She had been overwhelmed by stressors prior to this series of events. The sense of being overwhelmed by physical or emotional demands or by problems with life (those uncontrollable events) is usually a precursor of crisis behaviors. The sense of being overwhelmed and emotionally dysregulated compromised my client's decision-making skills. Often, when people are in crisis, they ignore intuitive knowing and attend more to events that relieve some of the emotional pain or stress. My client did this when she ignored a warning light in her head about the man and her daughter. Even though she met with me during this time and I came up with a plan, she did not implement the plan. This often happens with people when they are in crisis states. The person with BPD cannot figure out how to problem-solve and/or ignores the solutions to the problem. It is the ignoring that makes people judge them as wanting the crisis to continue or "loving" crisis. In fact, it is that they have the experience of being overwhelmed by the crisis (she couldn't get him to leave because he looked at her in a way that made her not follow through with the plan). They do not believe that they can solve the problem or carry out a plan of action.

*H*ow You Can Help during Unrelenting Crisis

If you have tried to help your loved one when she is in a crisis-generating state, you have probably been disappointed and frightened for her. Maybe you've tried to make a case about different decisions that your loved one could make and she assured you that she would do so. Then, in the moment, she made a different, more emotional and impulsive decision. It could be that you talked to your loved one as she was engaging in the impulsive behavior, such as on the phone as she was writing her resignation, and you could not get her to say that she would do anything differently.

You are watching the car wreck. You can see that the speed and the turns that your loved one is making in the car are going to lead inevitably to a crash. You are trying to help change the way she is driving the car, but she can't hear you. Or she can hear you but doesn't think she can do anything differently. As you watch, your loved one crashes and burns. You are angry, and you are so disheartened because different variations of the same behaviors come up over and over again.

Encourage Your Loved One to Get Professional Help

The good news is that these behavioral patterns are the ones that typically get people with BPD into treatment. The bad news is that they usually seek treatment after the crash and not before. You may do everything that you can, from physically intervening to talking yourself to death, before the crisis comes to a head, to no avail. When the final crisis hits, however, you have an opportunity to help your loved one by suggesting effective treatment for BPD. See Chapter 13 for descriptions of effective treatments and how to find practitioners who can provide them.

Take Every Opportunity to Help Your Loved One Regulate Emotion

Mark is exhibiting very poor judgment. He quit his job, he has met a woman that you, his adult child, do not approve of, and he plans to marry her. He is talking about moving to the Caribbean and making his living by playing in the casino every night. As he is making these decisions, you and the other people in his life are responding negatively— begging him to see reason, chastising him for being silly and irresponsible, appealing to his love by saying you can't stand being so worried about him, threatening not to see him or his wife-to-be if he follows through on these plans. Mark is becoming increasingly upset by these responses, and the interpersonal pressure is becoming overwhelming. His reaction is to tell you he will just stay in the States and kill himself. Meanwhile, he is selling his house and terminating his friendships. All the while, he is spending more and more time in bars and driving home after drinking each night. You're waiting for the worst to happen.

What could you and Mark's other relatives do differently? As painful as it is to hear, you may not be able to stop the speeding train that Mark is on. But you could, whenever you're confronted with one of his dubious decisions, apply the five-step response from Chapter 4. That is, do everything to regulate your own emotion so that you don't add to Mark's emotion. Second, ask him if he is overwhelmed, what is causing him to be overwhelmed, and how what he is doing or planning to do will manage the sense of being overwhelmed and then see if you can steer him toward brainstorming alternatives. Ask him if there are other ways he has answered the same need in the past. Help him go through the problem-solving steps in Chapter 7. If he's not open to exploring alternatives, at least you've done something to control your own emotion, which is to your benefit. Now you can take some extra measures to deal with the inevitable if Mark repeatedly proves closed to reconsidering his decisions and taking more beneficial measures to deal with his needs and desires in life.

Learn to Tolerate Your Own Distress

Watching someone you care deeply about heading for disaster is extremely distressing, so much so that many people will do anything to head off the catastrophe they see coming. Maybe you've loaned your loved one large sums of money to get him out of trouble even though you couldn't afford it. Perhaps you've paid legal fees, replaced wrecked cars, or paid for psychiatric care for someone without insurance. The problem with these decisions is that, even if they aren't actually impulsive ones, they can get you into your own unrelenting crisis. Not only is that not fair to you, but your preoccupation with your own problems can make you unavailable to help your loved one in nonmonetary ways. And if that happens, the crisis for both of you just might be unremitting for a long time. That's why I put learning to tolerate distress right at the top of the list of ways to help during your loved one's unrelenting crisis.

Tolerating distress involves regulation of your own emotions; see the ideas in Chapter 4. But don't just take measures to lower your emotions in the moment, like holding ice in your hand as described in Chapter 4. Also do some planning to incorporate ways to be good to yourself, to soothe yourself and cultivate calm every day, or at least as often as you can. Find mental and physical activities that let you focus on other things. We call this *distracting*. Do something that you can do mindfully (go to a movie, call a friend, work a puzzle). See if you can find some meaning in or something to learn from the distressing situation. Practice paced breathing (you can get this on YouTube). You are not going to solve the problem; you just have to get through the moment without doing something worse. In other words, you have to deal with being overwhelmed in the same way that we would want your loved one to deal with being overwhelmed.

> It's okay to put aside solving the problem and distract yourself to get through your own distress in this moment.

Look back at Chapter 4 and continue to practice acceptance. Remember that acceptance of what is will keep hopelessness from compounding your distress to the point where you feel like you just have to do *something*, whether it will really solve the problem at the center of the crisis and whether it's good for *you* or not.

And finally, you can use some of the ideas I suggest below to help your loved one avoid the impulsive behavior that lands him in crisis.

You can access your own wise mind during your loved one's crisis as well as finding ways to distract yourself so that distress doesn't overwhelm you.

Recognize Your Loved One's Capabilities

Distress and worry are not the only emotional reactions you're likely to have to unrelenting crisis. Many people alternate between fear about what will befall their loved one and fury over the chaos that keeps sucking them in. Often anger is the result of continually trying to advise your loved one on how to avoid crisis-generating behavior and having your advice ignored. Your advice is most likely to be ignored when *you* can see that your loved one is either in crisis or on the verge of it but she does not. Mark thought his decisions were sound because he became attached to a new woman who encouraged him to follow the path that his family knew would lead to disaster. Fear of being abandoned by this new girlfriend (and therefore deemed "worthless") kept Mark from seeing that he was making bad choices.

Like Bella, some people with BPD ask for advice when they are about to make an impulsive move. Act from the assumption that they want to hear your answer. If they don't take your advice, try not to judge. Sometimes people ask for advice because they want others to know or mind-read how bad they feel. Sometimes they want validation that they "deserve" to go on a cruise or that they are making a wise decision. Many times, the advice seems sound when the person with BPD is with you, but when you two are not together the stressors and emotions come back up and the crisis behaviors return.

Kathy met a man on the Internet who claimed to be a millionaire. He sent her pictures from "foreign countries" that usually showed him in a T-shirt that had the name of the country on it but were taken in a setting that could have been his own living room. She made plane reservations to go see him on several occasions, but he canceled at the last minute because he was supposed to be in a rain forest in South America that had no phone service (of course, he texted her from the same location). In one case she actually flew to his hometown and stayed in a hotel for several days until he told her that he was out of town on business.

When Kathy asked my opinion about the man, I told her that I was suspicious of anyone who joined a website that asked people if they were millionaires but didn't vet them and that I was concerned that she was purchasing flight tickets that he was then asking her to cancel. I asked her to consider the possibilities with me, and she could tell me that the man was, in all probability, a fraud. When she got back to her apartment, she was alone again and felt that she couldn't tolerate being alone. She continued to pursue him even after he told her he was married, because, to her, having a married man online was better than being alone. Many of the poor choices that people with BPD make in relationships are driven by inability to tolerate being alone.

Remember a couple of important suggestions from Chapter 8:

• *Don't assume your loved one is competent*—that he could have avoided causing this crisis. Kathy may have a good job and look in control, but she does not have the capacity to tolerate being alone, especially when other stressors compound her discomfort.

• *Balance intervening with coaching.* Constant intervention could leave you tapped out and in your own unrelenting crisis and won't help your loved one learn to solve problems without the impulsive actions that cause new crises. See if you can discern what your loved one's capabilities really are. If she simply can't stop invalidating herself, or no matter what measures you take to try to bring emotion down in individual moments she stays intensely emotional, find a time shortly after these encounters to stress the potential benefit of professional help. (Doing this in the heat of the moment probably will not be effective.) Also continue to practice acceptance of your loved one's inability to do certain things—anger will only exhaust your energy and erode your health faster than the crises at hand are already doing.

Sometimes the humane thing to do is to help your loved one by intervening. You might look at what the overwhelming stressors are and try to figure out a way to help with them. Maybe you could invite Bella to go to the beach for a weekend with you, instead of spending a lot of money on a cruise. A loved one might have asked my client if she could take my client's children to a movie to give her a break from the stressor. If you want to do something to help your loved one, look at where the stressors are and try to do something to help. If you do something to change the consequences of the crisis behavior later on, you may accidentally reinforce the crisis behavior. Think about the things that are making your loved one vulnerable to the crisis behaviors (loneliness, financial stress, physical problems) and make the intervention there.

Three Ways to Encourage Wisdom

People like Kathy, who are embroiled in a crisis they're not even aware of, will often ask for advice and then proceed to do what they would have done anyway. This is one of the routes by which they get into *unrelenting* crisis to begin with. As I've said, sometimes the only way to interrupt the cycle is to wait until the crash occurs and then do everything you can to get your loved one into treatment. That doesn't mean, however, that I think you should refuse to give your opinion when asked for it. It does mean that there are ways to respond to a request for advice that might have a more positive effect.

1. *Help your loved one access "wise mind."* What we in DBT call "wise mind" is the synthesis of emotion and reason. Wise mind can be used at any point, at the beginning of the crisis or as the crisis is building. It may seem that the goal is to get your loved one to leave emotion out of the picture and use only reason. This would be really difficult for an emotional person, and asking her to get rid of emotion in decision making could be so drastically invalidating that she would not consider the options that emerge. So, moving to a place where she asks herself to consider the emotions and the logical solution to a problem may be effective.

There are several ways to access wise mind. Most of them involve breathing and "listening" to the wisdom inside, as opposed to "thinking" about the problems. Try this practice to understand the difference: Breathe in and out. Don't change how you breathe to make it deeper; just breathe naturally. As you breathe, on the inhaled breath, ask yourself a question about something that may be troubling you. On the exhalation, listen for the answer. Don't think about the answer; just listen. Sometimes you may not hear anything. Keep doing it. Sooner or later, an answer will pop into your head and you will hear it. This is usually the wisdom of your solution. The problem, of course, is that we often know what the wise answer is and don't act on the wisdom. This is often the case with people with BPD. Remember, if your loved one chooses not to act on it, there may be nothing you can do other than to try to tolerate the distress you feel. But you can also try two other options:

2. *Do a pros and cons.* You saw an example of this technique in Chapter 4. The key to doing the pros and cons is to look at all sides of the problem. In the example with the client above, I would have her do

the pros of continuing to have contact with the man, the cons of continuing to have contact, the pros of stopping talking with him, and the cons of stopping talking with the man. At first, it may seem that the pros of continuing and the cons of stopping talking are the same. However, the lists will be different if they are complete. After it is finished, have your loved one step back and look at what the "wise" solution is. This is not a quantitative pros and cons, so don't count the answers; look for the ones with the most strength and wisdom. Here is an example of the pros and cons for Kathy and the married "millionaire":

	Staying in Contact	Stopping Contact
Pros	Have someone to talk to Not lonely Not bored He might leave his wife	Won't ruin his marriage No guilt Won't get hurt later Feel better about myself
Cons	Won't meet other men Get my heart broken by him Guilt about him being married Guilt about hurting him	No one to talk to No "buzz" from new man Will get lonely and bored

Although the lists are about the same length, if you ask which actions are wise, this pros and cons indicates that Kathy would be wiser to stop the contact.

3. *Simply ask what would be the wise thing to do.* If your loved one is in DBT, she'll be familiar with the terminology and you can ask, "What does your wise mind say?" Otherwise just ask, "What is the wise thing to do here?" It is amazing to me that people, even in the heat of emotion, can usually tell others what the wise decision is. Again, it is following the wisdom that is often hard for all of us.

Help Your Loved One Find Better Ways to Distract Himself

One reason that people with BPD find themselves in the middle of unrelenting crisis is that they have difficulty tolerating negative events in their lives. They're emotionally vulnerable to such events, and their history has taught them that they'll not only suffer pain in response to these events but also be told that their pain is unacceptable and shameful. So your loved one may know that a certain alternative would be the wise choice yet be unable to take that choice because it might trigger a negative event. Kathy might have to face being lonely. She might have to face the shame of having been fooled. When something difficult occurs, people with BPD want to escape or avoid the problem or the distressing emotion. We all have this impulse, actually. If your beloved pet dies, you might prefer not to grieve. After all, grieving hurts. But you go through it because you know you have to and that you'll survive. People with BPD think they will be overwhelmed by their grief; they truly believe they won't survive, and so they do whatever it takes to prevent themselves from grieving. Kathy might do the same in order to avoid feeling lonely or foolish.

I tell my clients that it's the urge to get away from the negative life events that's the problem, because so often their methods of getting relief are so problematic. The solution is pretty simple, though for people with BPD it requires a lot of practice: Find benign ways to distract yourself. We do a lot of things like this without really thinking about it:

- Read a book
- Go to a movie
- Watch TV
- Visit with a friend
- Do charity work
- Work Sudoku puzzles
- Knit
- Paint a room
- Clean your house

These are all possibilities you can suggest that your loved one get used to using to distract himself from negative events when he has the urge to escape. Tell your loved one to do anything that she knows she can do with all of her attention. Tell her to let the emotions settle down while she's distracting herself. This really works. The problem for people with BPD is that distracting themselves is not a long-term fix of the emotion. When your loved one stops distracting herself, the distress will often return in full force. Remind her that this may happen but that the purpose of distracting is to get temporary relief, just like going to the bar and getting drunk provides relief. The difference is that there are almost no negative consequences to painting a room or doing charity work.

In the long run, people with BPD have to learn how to actively solve problems. Distracting really only does temporarily relieve emotion. Many times, though, distracting and wise mind help to reduce emotion enough to enable problem solving. That's when you can help your loved one use the problem-solving strategies in Chapter 7.

The thing about unrelenting crisis is that it is not sustainable. People have to find some way to end the crisis. People with BPD will engage in a behavior that has the consequence of ending the crisis (a suicide attempt) or they will just shut down altogether. We call both of these *inhibited grieving*, the subject of the next chapter.

"Nothing's Wrong—I'm Fine"

You're confused by Sarah's reactions to things. There are times when she doesn't seem to experience the sadness in her life. Yet you know there are times when she's overwhelmed by despair over her life not being what she wants it to be. You can visibly see her shut down when you think she should be having emotions. She seems to bounce between having crisis after crisis and having no emotion at all.

Voluble expression of emotion is often a reflection of how overwhelming emotions can feel to people with BPD. But when someone has been feeling overwhelming emotions for years, sometimes a different kind of behavior emerges. Typically, those with BPD have experienced significant losses throughout life. Sometimes they lose people who matter to them. Often they lose their sense of control. The chaos that may characterize their lives can lead them to expect loss even where it hasn't occurred. So people like Sarah might feel they are suffering a loss whenever they feel criticized, dismissed, or trivialized. Whether loss is real or perceived, naturally they respond quite negatively. As the losses in their life accumulate over time, their experience is that their lives are full of sadness. Accumulated loss can have two different effects:

1. *People with BPD become sensitized to loss.* When we have a particular negative emotional reaction over and over, we usually become sensitized to the precipitating event. If every time you encountered a large black dog you ended up bitten, over time you'd find yourself instantly

179

and intensely afraid whenever you saw such a dog. The same thing happens to those with BPD when they believe they are experiencing a loss. Sensitivity leads your loved one to react strongly to real or perceived loss. She may not recover from the loss of a pet, even though most people eventually do. Or if she thought you should "have her back" in a particular situation but believes you didn't behave as if you did, she may respond as if she has suffered a terrible loss.

2. *People with BPD stop processing losses.* As losses accumulate, your loved one may become so overwhelmed by sadness that she ceases to process any losses. Her beloved pet dies or her marriage ends, and she has no emotional reaction to the loss. It's been found in research studies that people with BPD, like people with posttraumatic stress disorder, have often experienced multiple significant losses at an early age. But because of their innate emotional sensitivity, the young people who later develop BPD don't recover from those losses. Time and experience, along with poor decision making, tend to compound the loss and their resulting grief over time. The long-term pattern of grief and sadness becomes so overwhelming that they simply stop processing losses, instead avoiding experiencing the emotions at all.

*O*verwhelming Sadness plus Avoidance of Emotion

The problem is that people with BPD experience overwhelming sadness *and* avoid having the emotions. We all, including people with BPD, understand that the only way out of emotions is to have them. But people with BPD, due to their emotional sensitivity and the reality that they typically lead lives full of sadness and grief, are often afraid of emotions. Therefore they seek to escape having them. When the inevitable losses in life occur, people with BPD cannot tolerate the sadness of the loss, and their response is to avoid grieving. There will be times when the

> People with BPD often alternate between expressing extreme sadness and expressing no emotion at all when you know they are probably feeling grief.

first response to loss exhibited by your loved one is to appear emotionless. But often what you will see is your loved one alternating between extreme emotional arousal (crying, etc.) and extreme emotional avoidance (no expression at all).

You may see your loved one try to escape by engaging in impulsive behaviors, such as drinking, cutting, or running away. This is the pattern of unrelenting crisis described in the preceding chapter. Or he may escape by shutting down emotionally. The cycle between extreme emotional arousal and emotional shutdown occurs because, as explained earlier, suppressed emotion inevitably "explodes" when it does emerge. People with BPD pile one unexperienced loss on another and another. These emotions become more difficult to avoid over time and exacerbate other emotional experiencing, and the cycle builds.

The Belief That Negative Emotion Will Never End

Your loved one may resist experiencing distressing emotions because she believes the emotion will never end. When my stepfather died, I was really sad. However, I had experienced loss before. My father had died when I was 20 years old. Grieving my father's loss was very difficult, but I did mourn, and because I did so, the mourning ended. I learned that I could grieve without drowning in the grief. When my stepfather died, I had learned through experience that I could grieve and that the sadness wouldn't last forever, so I was willing to experience the sadness. People with BPD, however, don't have that experience. They *have* had the experience of being caught up in a tidal wave of emotion that threatened to drown them. The results of grief for them have seemed unending and catastrophic. In fact, people with BPD have often had the experience of grief never ending.

Many people with BPD tell me they feel like they are nothing but a mass of emotion inside. They see themselves as being a ball of emotional yarn. If they pull the thread of negative emotion, they are afraid that they will never be able to stop the emotion and their ball of yarn will totally unravel. I have had many clients with BPD tell me that if they ever started crying they would never stop. Sometimes they don't even need to begin experiencing a negative emotion to feel afraid that they will be drowned by it.

Because of their sensitivity to emotions, people with BPD learn at an early age that their emotions can easily become uncontrollable. Scientists studying the disorder have found that sadness and grieving feel particularly uncontrollable to them. That's why, when we teach people emotional regulation skills in DBT, we tell clients that the disorder can make them emotion-phobic, especially grief-phobic. For some people with BPD, any negative emotion can cause them to shut down. For others with BPD, it's mostly grief that causes the shutdown. In DBT, we call this shutdown *inhibited grieving.*

*H*ow Do You Recognize Inhibited Grieving?

If your loved one is avoiding emotion, there are several ways you might recognize inhibited grieving. As mentioned above, impulsive behavior is often one sign that a person is attempting to shut down emotions. Another way to recognize inhibited grieving is through lack of facial expression or body language that you would expect with that emotion.

Lack of Facial Expression and Emotional Body Language

A person who is inhibiting grieving will usually have a flat facial expression, and she won't express the emotion at all. You won't see any evidence of the emotions you would expect in a given situation—in the same way as you would have been perplexed by Sarah's apparent lack of emotion when you knew the circumstances of the moment were likely causing her to feel despair.

All emotions have hardwired physiological expressions associated with them. Those expressions are universal. If you take a kitten to a kindergarten in Ukraine, the emotions reflected on the faces of the children will be the same as they would be if you took the kitten to a kindergarten in Fiji. The children would smile. They would jump up and down. Their eyes would widen and sparkle. They would run toward you. The expression of their happiness would be apparent. You could label that emotion, and if you sat the children down, you could teach them to label it happiness. If you then took away that kitten, the kids in Ukraine and Fiji would again express their emotions in the same way: They might frown or cry. They would use words of sadness ("Oh, please, don't take him"). The children's faces would show sadness, eyes and mouths turning down. Sadness usually expresses itself with crying. The person's physiological arousal slows, so maybe the kids would slow down their motions, such as starting to drag their feet instead of leaping around. The point is that usually when a person is sad we can tell he is sad.

When your loved one is inhibiting grieving, she may show no emotion at all or may show an emotion that is not related to the experience. She will not communicate feeling the emotion. If you ask a person in

> One difference between inhibited grieving and apparent competence is that in the former the person doesn't express or acknowledge sadness at all where in the latter the person expresses sadness in words but doesn't show it nonverbally.

inhibited grieving what she's feeling in relation to a cue, she will say, "I am feeling nothing." She will not look sad, nor will she acknowledge sadness. This is different from apparent competence, where she would say, "I feel sad," but would not look or sound very sad. The treatment for inhibited grieving is for your loved one to *experience* sadness. The treatment for apparent competence is for your loved one to accurately *express* the sadness.

How People Attempt to Inhibit Grieving

People with BPD who shut down sadness and grief may try to avoid the emotions in two ways: by avoiding the internal experience of the emotion and by avoiding the external cues of the emotion.

Avoiding the Internal Experience of Emotion

When your loved one is inhibiting grieving, she may show no emotion at all. Or she may show an emotion that is not related to the experience—such as smiling when you know something that just happened would ordinarily make her sad. This reaction, discussed further below, is not the same as the incongruent or muted emotional expression discussed in Chapter 8. When a person with BPD is exhibiting apparent competence, she is probably having the experience of the emotion but is not outwardly showing it or accurately showing it. We call this *masking emotion*. In inhibited grieving, your loved one is not experiencing the emotion at all. Sometimes she may be aware that she's shutting down the sadness and grief, and sometimes it may be so automatic that she doesn't even realize she's avoiding the experience of the emotion.

Avoidance of the internal experience of emotion is usually not intentional. It's something that is learned over time. For many people, shutting down sadness becomes almost a reflex. If you have ever been talking with your loved one and suddenly her face goes flat, with no emotional expression, she may be inhibiting the emotion without being consciously aware of doing so.

Other times people with BPD avoid the internal experience of emotion intentionally. Your loved one can't stop her pet from dying, but when sadness wells up in her, she will immediately avoid it. I have had clients who have said, "I don't do sad. The minute I feel sad coming on, I shut it down." When people go out and get drunk so that they don't have to go home and be alone with an emotion, they are intentionally avoiding or inhibiting emotion.

Sometimes, however, a person with BPD who is not expressing the emotions that you would expect in a given situation is masking the emotion, as discussed in Chapter 8. She may show you a different emotion from what she is experiencing or she may show you nothing at all (like a judge in a television game show). How do you know the difference between masking emotion and avoiding it altogether? Think of the difference between a person who is "taking care of business" at the funeral of a beloved parent, not expressing sadness or loss, and the one who is either almost catatonic at the funeral or isn't even there—but out drinking at the nearest bar to avoid feeling the grief at all.

Dissociation

Sometimes your loved one will tell you that she is "fine" and that there is nothing wrong. Even at events like funerals when other people are expressing emotion, people with BPD will often inhibit the sadness and not look sad at all. That may be because people with BPD sometimes dissociate during inhibited grieving. Dissociation is basically the shutting down of emotion by separating consciousness from emotion. All of us dissociate. Daydreaming is a low form of dissociation. So is driving a familiar route on "autopilot" and not remembering your trip home from the grocery store, as I noted in Chapter 1. Our conscious mind kind of separates from our body and emotions for a little while. In severe dissociation, the person may continue to function or may actually just sit for hours and do nothing. What people are not doing when dissociating is experiencing the current moment. People who have been traumatized sometimes dissociate when they are in the presence of cues of the trauma.

There are many reasons for dissociation, but the important thing for you to know is that when people are "zoning" or "flat," they are not experiencing emotions. Of course, as mentioned earlier, these emotions often accumulate, unexperienced, and will erupt later into what can become extreme crisis. Often, people with BPD will engage in impulsive, high-risk behaviors to help them escape the emotions. As they vacillate between behaviors that are increasing the crisis and impulsive behaviors to help them avoid emotions, the emotions and the problems associated with them are escalating.

Shifting to Another Emotion

Sometimes people avoid one emotion by experiencing another. If you have ever been really sad and then gotten angry, did you notice whether the anger was more comfortable or manageable, for lack of a better word, than the sadness? You were learning that anger helps you avoid sadness. Now think about the person you care about with BPD when she's intensely angry. Sometimes the anger is related to the prompting event. Someone berates your sister without cause, and she gets angry. Many times, however, the anger functions to shut down other, uncomfortable emotions. It could be that your loved one has a problem at work and loses her job. Sadness at the loss of a job would be a completely understandable emotion. When she comes home and begins telling you about the emotion, she is very angry at all of her coworkers and supervisors. The anger could be primary to the job loss, but chances are the anger is functioning to keep your loved one from feeling the sadness of losing her job.

If you think your loved one is really experiencing sadness but is avoiding it with anger or another emotion, validate the sadness. Don't tell her she is actually experiencing sadness and showing anger. Doing so would invalidate her and probably lead to an explosion. Instead, say something like "If this happened to me, I would feel really sad" and observe the response. Sometimes normalizing will bring your loved one to the emotion. She may negate what you say by saying, "Well, that's you, but I am not sad. I am angry." Don't argue. If she seems open to what you're saying, talk about how scary and overwhelming sadness is. Tell her you will not leave her to drown in her sadness.

Avoiding the External Cues of Sadness

Your loved one may also avoid any external cue that brings up sadness if she is trying to inhibit grieving. The cues can be events that trigger sadness. Avoiding situations that trigger sadness may be your loved one's attempt to control the environment so that he is not in danger of experiencing any negative emotion. I had a client once who longed to have a relationship with her estranged father. In many ways, she suffered from not having a relationship with him. However, when he invited her to visit him, she always refused. Others in her life accused my client of "wanting to be miserable," but the reality was just the opposite. She was so afraid that the relationship might not work out and she would have to lose her father all over again that she could not get herself to visit him.

You may find that your loved one avoids places, people, and things that are associated with past sadness and loss. I had a client who would not go into a synagogue because her grandfather had been a rabbi and he had died. Because she did not want to experience the understandable sadness that would arise in her when she saw a rabbi in the synagogue, she quit attending. Not attending services caused the client to be more isolated and to feel even more sadness, guilt (from avoiding her religious observances), and shame. Those emotions then had to be avoided, so she began to drink on Friday nights when her family would be sitting down to Shabbat dinner, and she drank until Saturday night when her religious week ended. When my client's family tried to talk to her about what was going on, she would respond with a blank expression and not speak. Her mother thought she was being petulant and uncooperative. The reality was that she was avoiding the emotions that she was feeling. She was in a cycle of avoiding environmental cues to her sadness, which caused more negative emotion that she had to avoid, which raised questions from her family, which caused more negative emotions that she had to avoid. And the cycle continued. Of course, this cycle could not go on forever. Her family came to see her to try to find out what was going on, and she locked herself into the bedroom, took an overdose, and ended up in the intensive care unit of the local hospital.

*W*hat to Do about Inhibited Grieving

As a family member, you will probably not be able to "treat" your loved one's inhibited grieving. If your loved one is shutting down, validation is your best strategy.

Validate the Emotion Your Loved One Is Likely to Be Experiencing—and How Tough It Is to Feel It

Validate the emotions that she must be experiencing and validate how hard it is to experience them. In DBT we recognize that extreme emotional reactions by therapists can push the person with BPD from one extreme to the other. This idea can be applied to those who love people with BPD too. So, if your loved one is going through a divorce and you can see that she is not feeling the sadness required to deal with the loss and is drinking every night, you have to moderate your own emotional reaction. If you get extremely sad for your loved one and express this to her, she may do something really impulsive to avoid the emotion and perpetuate the crisis. On the other hand, if you don't react to her situation with a "real" sadness, you will invalidate her experience of sadness and/or she will think she is overreacting and move to impulsivity and self-invalidation.

Generate Hope

The second thing to do is to generate hope for your loved one that she can survive the current sadness she is experiencing. Whatever loss is precipitating the current crisis can be survived. If your loved one is willing, you can offer solutions for re-creating her life in the present in a way that acknowledges what was lost. Say something like "I know that it feels like nothing has been the same since your marriage ended. It's not. Your life is really different. Can I help you figure out some things that you can do right now to start a new life and still respect your old life?" *Remember the five-step process laid out in Chapter 4.* If your

> You can be the keeper of hope for a person who thinks her sadness will never end.

loved one begins to grieve openly with you, help her have the emotion without avoiding it. If the grief is over the loss of a person, have her relate her memories to you while experiencing the emotion. If she starts to shut down, ask her what she is feeling in her body. **Emotions are physical sensations. If you want to experience an emotion, ask yourself what you're feeling in your body and pay attention to the sensations.**

Accept Your Own Sense of Relief at the Lack of Emotional Expression

Sometimes, when your loved one has been in a perpetual state of crisis, it's easy to feel some relief when she shuts down all of the emotion. Acknowledge to yourself the relief that you're experiencing. However, it's important to understand that inhibiting emotion is not an effective coping skill for any of us and that it is a place born of misery in our loved ones.

Look for Exposure Therapy

The only way to overcome the inhibited grief is to actually experience emotions. But as you've learned, people with BPD will avoid events that trigger emotions as well as the emotions themselves. Behavior therapy offers a technique called *exposure* (to emotional cues) that can help the person with BPD experience rather than avoid emotions like sadness and grief. Exposure is a sophisticated, difficult technique, and I will not try to teach it to you. If your loved one has had trauma in his life, it would be beneficial to get him into therapy with a person trained in exposure treatments.

Understand, however, that having someone experience emotion is not the same as "getting it out." I often hear television psychologists tell people that they need to "get it all out" as if the emotion is an "it" that is imprisoned somewhere inside of the person and that it must be set free. As a behaviorist, this is not what I believe. There is no evidence that regurgitating all of the sadnesses of anyone's past ever made the person feel better. *In fact, doing this can make people with BPD worse and can lead to an increase in suicidal behaviors.* The ultimate goal is to help your loved one fully experience emotions as they come up in her life so that they do not accumulate and cause her more misery in the long run. Offer validation, express hope, forgive yourself for being relieved at getting a break from expression of intense emotion, and see if you can get your loved one some professional help. In Part III you'll find help dealing with your own emotions and then with finding that professional help that can make a difference.

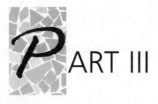

PART III

Dealing with Crisis
and Getting Help

Handling Your Own
Difficult Emotions

In any relationship, we experience the full gamut of emotions. Loved ones of people with BPD often report that they experience intense emotions in dealing with the parent, child, sibling, or spouse with BPD. The transactions that occur between people intensify or dilute depending on the interaction and the arousal of emotion. If your coworker is upset with you and says something harsh, you'll probably have an emotional reaction, and that experience will make your next interaction with that coworker different than it would have been otherwise: Maybe you'll be more wary than you used to be and ready to react with anger or defensiveness. You might even be emotionally sensitive or reactive in your very next encounter with someone else, even though that person had nothing to do with the original emotion-arousing incident. These transactions develop until, usually, the workday ends and we all start over the next day. None of us operates in a vacuum.

Think about a time when your loved one was really emotional. When she was emotionally aroused, did your emotional arousal intensify also? If she was angry, did you get angry in response? If so, your anger of course increased her arousal, thus increasing your arousal, and so on. What about afterward? Did you feel angry at yourself or at her? Did you feel guilty about your behavior or, if you are a parent, guilty about things that you did in the past that you think may have contributed to your loved one's current problems or diagnosis of BPD? Maybe you were afraid that you said or did something that caused your loved one's destructive behavior or a suicide attempt. It could be that you were filled with despair and sadness about how your loved one's life, and yours in turn, has not turned out the way you envisioned.

It's perfectly normal to have a range of emotions when you're involved with someone who is really suffering. If your loved one had a terminal illness, you probably would accept that range of emotions, but our culture makes normalizing behavior more difficult when dealing with people with mental illness and behavioral disorders. I discussed anger and sadness earlier in the book because they so often factor into the individual interactions with a person who has BPD and the immediate aftermath of those interactions—and because unregulated anger can be so damaging to both of you in the moment and later. In Chapter 4 I described how you could use compassion, acceptance, and the skill called *opposite action* to deal with these normal responses. But when you have cared about someone with BPD for a long time, there are other emotions that tend to lurk in the background and build, especially when you have been dealing with crisis after crisis and feel despair over where it will all end. Those emotions are guilt, fear, and despair, and they're the subject of this chapter.

> It's just as normal to have a range of emotions when a loved one has a behavioral disorder as it is when someone you care about has a serious physical illness.

The Pitfall of Unexamined Guilt

Guilt, by definition, is the emotion that we experience when we have engaged in a behavior that violates our own moral code(s) or values. Guilt makes you want to make reparations for the harm you've done; repairing is the action of the emotion called guilt. If a child upsets his mother, he will draw a picture or bring her a flower to make things better. If you step on someone's foot in a department store, you'll have a moment of guilt that leads you to repair, or say "I'm sorry" to the person whose foot you may have hurt. Guilt keeps us from doing things that hurt others and, when proportionate to our behavior and circumstances, is a very important, effective emotion.

People with BPD often have out-of-control guilt. They either feel guilty about everything, absorbing all of the hurts and wrongs in the world and believing they caused them—my experience most of the time with BPD—or feel guilty about very few things, not understanding the pain they cause others. Part of therapy with people with BPD is aimed at getting them to understand their guilt, which decreases self-loathing and self-invalidation. If your loved one is in therapy, chances are she is doing work on guilt and its first cousin, shame, which has been discussed at length earlier in the book.

Guilt is as prevalent in the loved ones of those with BPD as it is in the person who has the disorder. And it can be just as harmful, mainly because it often goes unexamined. When you feel guilty, you may try to make reparations without thinking, as automatically as you would if you stepped on someone's foot in a store. Or, if the guilt you feel immediately makes you feel shame, you might try to smother the guilt, moving forward without taking any repairing actions. Both of these responses can be problematic in dealing with a person who has BPD.

Guilt can be divided into two types: justified and unjustified guilt. If guilt remains unexamined, you won't know which you're feeling, and it's important that you do because that determines how you are likely to respond. If your guilt is unjustified and yet you act as if it's justified, you may try to make reparations that aren't helpful for you. If your guilt turns out to be justified but you don't try to repair, you may be missing a chance to change the transactions with your loved one in a positive way.

It may not seem easy to tell whether guilt is justified, but when you can define the difference between justified and unjustified guilt, it's not difficult to examine the guilt you feel to figure out which it is. Justified guilt is the guilt that emerges when you have engaged in a behavior that violates your values or morals. So, if you miss a lunch date with a friend, and one of your values is that you don't stand people up for appointments, you may feel justified guilt. So how do you recognize unjustified guilt? Think of this guilt as unfounded guilt—guilt you feel even though you didn't do anything that violates your values or ethics.

Trying to Make Reparations When None Are Needed

I've seen many people who love someone with BPD act on unjustified guilt, to the detriment of themselves, the person with BPD, and their relationship. Have you ever tried to make things better or make up for some perceived offense against your loved one with BPD? Maybe you did something that is effective and within your morals, but you still ended up feeling guilty. Let's say your daughter calls you at 11:00 P.M. on a Wednesday night and she is drunk. She says she wants to talk to you about her childhood, but she is rambling and demonstrates the emotionality that comes with intoxication. You communicate your limits and hang up the phone. Then you feel guilty for having done so. You think about how lonely she is, how emotional she is, and how you "owe" it to her to talk about her childhood. In response to that guilt, you may do two things:

1. You might call her back and talk with her even though she probably won't remember the conversation the next day (and, of course calling her will reinforce "drinking and dialing").
2. The next time she needs something that you probably would not provide, you give it to her even if you know it's not wise or helpful to her to do so. You're acting out of unjustified guilt.

I once worked with a woman who had a fight with her husband, then went into the bathroom to get away from the fight and take a bath—a response that I would call *functional behavior* because it's a positive, helpful way to respond to an upsetting event. When she was in the bathroom, however, she opened up the cabinet to get bubble bath and saw the ibuprofen. She took an overdose of the ibuprofen and ended up in the psychiatric hospital. During the hospitalization, she and her husband had a couple therapy session, and my client told her husband she never would have overdosed if they hadn't been fighting.

> *Unjustified guilt makes your behavior with your loved one ineffective, but the guilt just stays around, getting in the way of your decision making and torturing you.*

When she was discharged from the hospital, she came home to a dozen roses, and her husband fixed dinner and cleaned the house every day for several days. Eventually, of course, things went back to normal. Her husband quit cleaning and cooking and the roses wilted. The next time that my client and her husband had a disagreement, she went to the bathroom and took an overdose. Again, her husband bought flowers and changed his behavior. When I asked him why he did this, he said that he felt guilty about his wife being hospitalized. He believed it was his fault and he had to make things better. I asked him if he felt guilty about the disagreement. He said that he knew disagreements were a part of any relationship and that he had not yelled, cursed, or threatened her in any way (she corroborated this claim). He did not really feel guilty about the argument but felt guilty about the resulting hospitalization.

I helped him see that his guilt was unjustified and that his behaviors that came from the unjustified guilt (roses, cooking, cleaning) were actually functioning to reinforce his wife's behavior and increase her suicidality and hospitalizations. We worked it out so that if he said something during an argument that he felt guilty about, he would repair by apologizing, but that if she overdosed he would not buy flowers or change his behavior when his wife was discharged from the hospital. Doing this was difficult for the husband. He did feel bad when she was hospitalized. We had to set him up with another therapist to coach him on not buying flowers and tolerating his own guilt about not trying to make things "right" in the short term. A lot of the work focused on seeing that his behavioral change might make things "right" in the long term. We worked on the husband experiencing other emotions about the behavior—sadness, fear, frustration—and on noticing the guilty feelings and reminding himself that his behavior was not the cause of the suicide attempts. He had to tolerate the hospitalization without engaging in the repair behaviors, but over time his wife stopped overdosing and being hospitalized.

An important point to keep in mind about reinforcers, as explained earlier in the book, is that the fact that the husband's behavior was reinforcing my client's suicidal behavior does not mean that she was *deliberately* attempting suicide to get the roses and changes in her husband's behavior. Often, reinforcers work without our being aware of their effect. Until my client and her husband figured out the reinforcers, neither one of them knew that they were at work on the behavior. That's how reinforcers work. Sometimes we know what they are (we work to get paid), and sometimes we don't.

Is Your Guilt Justified?

The man just described was experiencing unjustified guilt over his wife's suicidal behavior. It wasn't that hard for him to determine that he hadn't done anything to violate his values. To examine your own guilt, simply ask yourself if your behavior has violated your values. If you find it hard to articulate your values or morals, do some research. If you espouse a religion or spiritual practice, look at the "do's and don'ts" of your religion. If you don't practice a religion, you can search the Internet for moral codes and find websites that will help you decide what your values really are. There is a very interesting website named *www. universalbehaviorcode.com* that lists ten realms of moral behavior that include things like doing no harm, loving your family, and respecting others. Most value systems, whether attached to a religious practice or not, have commonalities that involve looking at the negative consequences of behavior so as not to harm others.

Most of you won't need to bone up on morals and values to figure out what yours are, however. In DBT (introduced earlier and discussed more fully in Chapter 13), we teach our clients a concept we call *wise mind*, which is a capacity for wisdom that we can all tap into instinctually. In Chapter 9 I recommended ways that you could encourage your loved one to consult her wise mind so that her decisions wouldn't be as likely to lead to crisis. To access wise mind yourself, breathe in, ask, "Have I done something that is against my values," and listen. Do this until you have the answer. Even therapists being trained in DBT are surprised to discover that people with BPD can answer accurately and easily when they ask themselves what their wise-mind values are. So can you.

How to Respond to Unjustified Guilt

If you notice that you're feeling guilty and then ascertain that it's unjustified, what do you do if that determination doesn't make the guilt evaporate? The way to make your guilt subside is to engage repeatedly in the behavior that is triggering the guilt—or, in the case of the husband above, *not* engage in the behavior over and over again. If you don't expose yourself over and over to what results in guilt for you, the guilt will sustain itself. The husband in the preceding story had to resist making unjustified reparations repeatedly before his mind registered the fact that he could tolerate his wife's suicidality without trying to "fix" it with flowers, dinner, and housecleaning. It wasn't easy, of course, because when he stopped responding with those "reparations," his guilt increased dramatically for a while. We've talked about the phenomenon that psychologists call an *extinction burst* before—that when you change a behavior meant to reverse or reduce an emotion you don't want to feel, the emotion is going to increase before it decreases. It's your brain's way of upping the volume on a signal that you used to heed at a lower volume. It's only when you continue to ignore the urge to engage in the behavior that the emotion starts to recede. If you don't do this, your guilt will not dissipate and you will not be effective in your relationship with your loved one. If instead you obey the louder signal and engage in your repairing behavior (buy flowers) when your guilt is in that heightened stage, you will reinforce your own guilt and make it harder for you to lower it. It's hard to ignore the insistent signal of an even more uncomfortable level of guilt, but remember that the increase is part of a wave and the guilt will go up but it *will* come down.

While training correctional officers in using this concept, I asked for an example, and the lieutenant, who was a former sergeant major and the picture of decorum and consistency in the prison, said that he wanted to be able to watch college football on Saturdays in the fall but felt guilty when he did so. We talked about the guilt being justified or unjustified, and he said that his guilt about watching games on Saturday was unjustified. He worked hard all week, and he did his chores at home before the games. There was no reason for him to feel guilty. I told him that the way to get the guilt to go away was to watch football every Saturday until it went down. I told him that when he originally sat down to watch football, he would feel the guilt go way up and he would have an urge to stop watching football but that he *must* keep watching. By the end of the season, his guilt was gone. I ran into him a few years later, and he told me that he can still watch football without feeling guilty.

Of course, treating guilt when dealing with your loved one is harder than watching college football. Part of the reason that this is true is that fear enters into the picture. Think of the last time you did something for your loved one that you intuitively knew was not helpful, either in the short term or in the long term. Was guilt a part of why you did it? If you tried to block your actions, what would happen next? Would you be afraid that your loved one might attempt suicide or end up in a hospital or start using again? You can get caught up in a cycle of fear and guilt, guilt and fear that will wear you out and ultimately can make your loved one worse. These two emotions can be so tightly intertwined that I'll talk about fear later in this chapter.

Parental Susceptibility

Parents and others who were involved in rearing children who grew up to struggle with BPD often feel like the disorder was their fault. Before you read another word, I want you to know that I do not think you are culpable for your loved one's BPD. To me, BPD is the perfect storm of variables—biology, goodness of fit, and a lot of factors that contribute to the development of a disorder. You can't say that your child's struggles are your fault; it does no one any good to ascribe blame. If you're not convinced of this, go back to Chapter 2 and review how BPD is believed to develop. It's very complicated. Many people who developed BPD grew up with perfectly nice, normal families who never intended anything but the best for their children. Somehow, though, many of us can't help believing that if there's something "wrong" with our kids it must be our fault. As scientists learn more about the neurobiology, or brain development, of people with BPD, we believe the physiological hardwiring is really important and that it is the fit between the biology and the environment that is key. Remember also that we all do things that are invalidating of others although it is not our intent. We don't know if your loved one would have developed BPD if you had done everything differently, or even a few things. We work really hard with your loved ones to get them to accept that their parents/caregivers really did the best that they were able with the child-rearing tools that they had.

You might feel like it can never hurt to err on the side of generosity in making up for any wrongs done to your son or daughter (or grandson or granddaughter if you raised your child's kids). Maybe you believe it makes you feel better to do whatever is in your power to do—just in case it will help your offspring. But one big problem with making reparations where none are due is that it can end up making you less effective in dealing with your relative. It may even hold your child back from overcoming some of the effects of BPD.

Sometimes family members spend their lives trying to repair the harm that they have done to their loved one in the past. All of us have done things that have hurt others. Most often the hurt was not intentional, and acting from guilt without realizing that it, and not wisdom, is driving our behavior is problematic. I have seen parents give their children money, cars, and rent or pay for multiple hospitalizations because they feel bad about things they did when their loved ones were young. They try to "fix" their adolescent or adult children because of their own guilt. There are times when helping out is really effective, but as I've said elsewhere in this book, being overly helpful can cripple your loved one and reinforce his sense of inadequacy. Loved ones who suffer from guilt will often intervene on behalf of the person with BPD and inadvertently reinforce suicidal or other problem behavior.

Liz came from a very affluent family. When she was a child, she had a younger brother who had brain cancer. Of course, much of their family's financial and emotional support was poured into the care of their son. Liz spent a great deal of her childhood alone as her parents took her brother to hospitals in the northeastern United States. As an adult, she had few emotional regulation or interpersonal skills and was chronically suicidal. She spent much of her 20s in private psychiatric hospitals. Liz would be discharged from the hospital, and her parents would set her up in a beautiful condo or apartment. Then they would require that she get a job and continue with therapy. Ultimately, because of Liz's extreme emotional vulnerabilities, she would lose her job and/or quit therapy. Her parents would keep paying for her beautiful living situation. Liz would become increasingly depressed and, finally, there would be another suicide attempt and hospitalization.

Many therapists had told her parents that they had to stop setting contingencies that they did not meet. However, they were unable to do so because they felt so guilty about not being present while Liz was growing up. They were trying to assuage their guilt and trying to make Liz's life better, but neither was happening. Instead, they were inadvertently making Liz worse, and their guilt was growing. Liz's parents knew they were not being helpful to her, but their guilt interfered with effective behavior. Eventually, we had a family session. In it, Liz's parents told her what they felt they had done that hurt her as a child and as an adult. They did not say that they should not have cared for their son (because that would have been unreasonable), but they apologized for the circumstances and for not finding a way to be with Liz more or to have Liz with them when they were in the Northeast. Then they told her that they were feeling guilt because of their current contribution to her increasing suicidal behavior.

> *Unjustified guilt compromises your effectiveness in trying to help your loved one change.*

Together, Liz and her parents worked to come up with manageable contingencies. Her parents gave her an allowance each month that would support a less luxurious apartment and basic necessities. To have more comforts, Liz had to work. They also told her that they would not pay for any more private hospitals but that they would pay for a good therapist. If she were to be hospitalized again, she would have to go to the local public hospital or, if she was working and had insurance, whatever hospital her insurance provided. She would have to pay the copayment for the hospitalization. To my knowledge, Liz has never been hospitalized again. She did have a period of time when she struggled with jobs and finances, but her parents held true to their word. When their guilt was manageable, so were the contingencies around Liz's behavior.

You may have noticed in the preceding story that the parents and I (and Liz) all agreed that their guilt was justified. The harm that was done to Liz by their absence wasn't *intentional*, but harm was definitely done. What was problematic for Liz's parents was not that they were making reparations out of unjustified guilt to begin with but that they felt guilt that *was* justified whenever Liz didn't uphold her part of the bargain and they were faced with imposing the consequences established.

What If Your Guilt Is Justified?

As with Liz's parents, most guilt that you're likely to decide is justified is still for unintentional harm. Reminding yourself of that may bring your guilt down just enough for you to tolerate making the appropriate repairs rather than going over the top as Liz's parents did. If you decide that some of your behaviors violated your values and harmed your loved one in some way, the next step is to determine what harm was done. If you stepped on the person's foot in the department store, the harm that was done was that you hurt the person's foot. If you discounted your loved one's emotional sensitivity when she was a child, you might have said things like "Stop that crying. You have nothing to cry about" or "You just need to stop wearing your heart on your sleeve." What harm did this do to your child? Did it make her feel like her emotions were wrong or that there was something wrong with her because she did cry? Think specifically about what you did and what the intended and (in most cases) unintended consequences were of your behavior. To sort out guilt, it's important to know the difference because it can allow you to make repairs without being overwhelmed by guilt for consequences you never intended or to avoid making repairs that were never warranted to begin with. The man who changed his behavior when his wife overdosed was acting on unjustified guilt, and he was able to stop changing his behavior once he realized that his actions had the unintended consequence of reinforcing her suicidal behavior. Liz's parents intended to help their ill son; they never intended to hurt their daughter. It was this realization that helped them stick to the contingencies they had set with her as an adult. Parents of an inconsolable child might tell her that she shouldn't cry because they want her to stop crying in that moment, and they want to relieve their own emotions and reestablish calm in the household. They don't intend for the child to end up without emotional regulation skills or to impart the belief that crying is wrong or weak. If you're afraid that your parenting had such unintended consequences, reminding yourself that they were unintended can help you apologize for those consequences.

> *Even justified guilt is often excessive if you don't remind yourself that you never intended to cause harm.*

Once you are clear about the behavior that is causing the "justified" guilt, or guilt that violates your values, make a repair. For most behaviors that occurred in the past, repairing requires telling your loved one what you did and what you see as the consequences, and apologizing for your behavior. Sometimes there is something you can do to make the repair, but for behaviors long past, often all you can do is apologize.

Finally, allow your loved one to have a response to your repair. In DBT we call this "accepting the consequences gracefully." Your loved one may get mad at you or may say that an apology is not enough. It may not be enough for her, but if you have done all you can do, it may be enough to make your guilt diminish. The next step is to let it go.

Susan held her daughter back a year prior to beginning the first grade. At the time, she had really good reasons for doing so. She thought that her husband was going to be transferred and they would be moving to another state. Ultimately, they didn't move and the daughter ended up being physically larger than the other children in her first-grade class the next year, where the other children made fun of her (an unintended consequence). Susan had always felt guilty about the decision and decided that her guilt was justified in that she had inadvertently caused harm to her daughter. *Take note: the fact that it was inadvertent is important.*

One day when Susan and her daughter were talking about something related to her schooling, Susan explained how she had made the decision and said she was sorry if keeping her daughter back had caused her problems later. The daughter had a big emotional reaction and told her mother all the ways that that one decision had affected her. I worked with Susan on realizing that she had made as much of a repair as she could make, and we decided on ways to validate the daughter about her experience but I encouraged her to let go of her guilt. This was a process. If the daughter had not had the intense emotional reaction she had, chances are that Susan's guilt would have decreased immediately. Instead, when the daughter brought the decision up again, her guilt would reignite, but Susan didn't want to continue apologizing because she thought it would reinforce her daughter's emotionality. So, she would validate her daughter's position, remind herself that she had apologized, and work on letting her own emotion go. After many efforts, Susan noticed that when her daughter told her that she was a bad mother for holding her back, she no longer felt guilty.

I am not advocating that you sit down and have a long discussion with your loved one and detail anything that may have happened over the years that you feel guilty about. People with BPD can be overwhelmed by that level of emotional conversation. At the same time, don't treat your loved one as if he is fragile. If there is a recurring theme in your relationship and it causes you to feel justified guilt, make the repair. People with BPD often tell their loved ones the things that they think their family "did wrong" in their lives. Unfortunately, the tone of the conversation can often be accusatory, and loved ones inevitably get on the defensive.

However, I have found that if family members can stay regulated (see Chapter 4) and have the discussion, the benefits to both parties— validation for the person with BPD and a decrease in guilt for the family members—are immense. I have also found, experientially, that if the person with BPD tells a loved one of a memory, emotion, or experience and it is completely negated ("That didn't happen") or trivialized ("Why are you making such a big deal out of this?"), the consequences for the person with BPD are often an increase in emotion and suicidality.

Alternately, remember from Chapter 3 that you don't want to validate the invalid. I once had a memory of something my mother had told me when I was around 6 years old. As things do with young minds and time, the memory became very convoluted. Finally, when I was in my 20s, I asked my mother why she had told me such a wild story and explained what she had told me. She was astounded. Of course she had never said anything like what I thought she had said. She felt terrible that I had carried her words around for a long time. What she didn't do was completely negate what I told her. She explained her memory of the event, and the reason for what she had been trying to tell her 6-year-old daughter—and validated how frightening my understanding of what she had said to me must have been. The acknowledgment of what I thought I had heard and its consequences for me soothed me and kept my mother from feeling guilty about her behavior.

How to Address Guilt Effectively

1. List the behaviors that are causing you to feel guilt.

2. Determine whether the things you did violated your values.

3. If they did violate your values or morals, describe them specifically.

4. List the intended and unintended consequences of your behavior for your loved one.

5. Make a repair for the behavior if guilt is justified.

6. Allow your loved one to have reactions to the repair.

Living with Fear

If you love someone with BPD, I don't have to explain what fear is. Fear can range from low-level worry ("Is he working today?" "Is he having urges to use?") to extreme, overwhelming fear ("Is he dead?" "Is he somewhere about to kill himself?"). For the sake of this discussion, I'm going to use the words *fear*, *worry*, and *anxiety* synonymously because they stem from the same primary emotion: fear. There are periods of time with your loved one when you may not have intense fear and other times when you're waiting for the phone to ring with horrific news. The problem with fear is that it can make you physically sick and that it can make you ineffective.

Soothe Yourself

One way to manage your susceptibility to fear is to use the self-care skills described earlier in this book. Researchers are continuing to find the negative effects of sustained anxiety: increases in cortisol, glucose, and adrenaline. These chemicals, if secreted over a sustained period of time, can cause gastrointestinal problems, heart problems, diabetes, obesity, adrenal problems, and pituitary problems. Fear and anxiety wear on you. I know it's hard to tell yourself not to worry or be afraid when it seems that your loved one is hanging on for dear life. Of course you're going to worry. The key is to treat your body with soothing, calming, and the skills discussed in Chapter 4 on a daily basis to counteract the effects of the anxiety.

Unmanaged Fear Leads to Avoidance

In addition to the physical reactions to ongoing fear/anxiety, these emotions can make you ineffective in dealing with your loved one. Fear, by definition, makes you want to avoid or get away from the thing that makes you fearful. Sometimes fear literally makes you avoid your loved one. I have known many family members who have stopped having relationships with their loved one with BPD because they could not tolerate the uncertainty of being involved with the person. They understood that their loved one was figuratively (and sometimes literally) standing on the ledge, but they could not tolerate the anxiety of feeling like they were on the ledge with their loved one. You may ultimately decide this for yourself, and if that is the case, I certainly will not judge you for doing so. There are occasions when family members are so affected physically (they develop the physical problems listed above) and worn out emotionally that they either have to take a break from the relationship or have to exit. If at all possible, I recommend taking a break (we call it a vacation) from the relationship over ending the relationship. I have known someone personally for a long time who has BPD and binge drinks. We recently went through a period of time when she was drinking and calling me and people I had introduced her to and crying or cursing at us on the phone. I realized that I needed a break from the relationship. The purpose of the vacation from the relationship is to keep the relationship from ending, which it may well do if her drinking and dialing behaviors don't stop. I followed the steps below. She was very hurt and upset with me for taking a break. She did not agree to stop drinking. She asked when I would be back. I told her that I would call her when a period of time went by without her calling me after drinking and when I felt comfortable being with her again. I assured her of my affection for her, validated that the break hurt her feelings, and expressed hope for our relationship in the future. I can only do this so many times before the relationship will end, but I am taking the break in the hope of saving the relationship.

If you're considering taking a break from the relationship, you may, as we discussed earlier, need to do a pros and cons about the relationship and examine your values to determine whether you will experience justified guilt for whatever steps you decide to take in the relationship.

Behaving Ineffectively Out of Fear

Fear can drive your behavior in spite of your best intentions. If you find yourself doing things that you know are ineffective, ask yourself what emotion you are experiencing right before you engage in the behavior. Often we do ineffective things out of fear. Family members capitulate to their loved ones because they are afraid of what will happen if they don't. Lily had a conflicted relationship with her partner, Mona, who had BPD. Lily wanted the relationship to work but was concerned that the relationship was in jeopardy because Mona was using drugs and cutting herself regularly. Mona would get emotionally upset and tell Lily that she should stay home from work and take care of her. Lily did not want to take time off and was in danger of losing her job because of too many absences. However, when she started to get ready to go to work while Mona was upset, her fear of what Mona would do while she was at work increased with every moment. Lily could not tolerate that fear and would stay home, not because she wanted to be with Mona but because staying home would assuage the fear. Fear made her avoid going to work and allowing her loved one to be alone.

Lily was very clear with me that she knew that staying home was reinforcing Mona's increased emotionality, but she could not manage the fear. Of course, I could not assure her that Mona would not use or cut while she was at work. I could assure her that over time Mona would cut more and use more if Lily stayed home. What needed to happen was

---

Deciding to Take a Break or Terminate the Relationship

1. Do a pros and cons (take a break vs. don't take a break, take a break vs. end the relationship, end the relationship vs. don't end the relationship) using the chart shown in Chapter 4.

2. Communicate the break or ending. If possible, give your loved one a chance to change her behavior ("If _____ doesn't change, I will need to take a break").

3. Recognize and tell your loved one that this is in your best interest and not necessarily hers.

4. With breaks, express hope that the relationship will get better.

5. Tell your loved one how you will know when the break is over.

---

for Lily to go to work over and over. If Mona did cut or use, the two of them would have to tolerate the outcome. I felt sure that over time the cutting and the drugging would go down if it was not reinforced by Lily's staying home. I also knew that every time Mona did not cut or drug, Lily's fear would decrease a little. My hypothesis was that both problem behaviors and the fear would decrease gradually.

Taking Care of Your Fear by "Taking Care" of Your Loved One

One sure way to get fear to subside temporarily is to attempt to control or fix everything for the person with BPD. Family members take over and try to manage the lives of the people with BPD. I've seen the loved ones of clients remove all of the knives from the house, put locks on cabinets, take over bank accounts, call their loved one and wake him up in the morning. They engage in all kinds of behaviors because they are afraid of what will happen if they don't do so. They "take care" of their loved ones and their fear at the same time.

There are several problems with this approach. If you manage the person with BPD without a plan and a timeline for transitioning away from the management—such as dispensing medications to a person who has been hospitalized following an overdose for only a short time, until she is more regulated—you will always be managing her. Taking care of your loved one will reinforce her own experience of not being able to take care of herself. Finally, your anxiety will never get relief. The only way for your anxiety to go down is for you to let go and for your brain to learn that the catastrophe you fear does not happen. As we discuss in Chapter 12, if you believe, in your wisest, less emotional place, that your loved one is at acute risk, then the threat of harm is real and present. At that point, you intervene on her behalf and do whatever is needed for her to stay alive. The problem is that this will reinforce your anxiety and make it stronger. As her risk comes down, you will have to begin treating it over again.

The Cycle of Fear and Guilt

Fear and guilt begin to cycle when you stop trying to control your loved one's life or fix all of her problems. Knowing that you and your loved one will benefit from some or all of your interventions provides little relief when you are anxious about the consequences of removing attention, money, or other assistance. Then, when you do stop taking the calls at 3:00 A.M., your loved one has an emotional reaction. Because of her reaction, your guilt emerges. Even though you know your guilt is not justified, you are afraid of the intensity of her emotional reaction, so you take the call. Now you feel guilt because you didn't do what you knew you needed to do and you're afraid that you're reinforcing crisis behavior. And the cycle continues. It continues because we think of people with BPD as being too fragile to tolerate what will change their learning. Your history with your loved one can also make you fearful of communicating limits or changing your own behavior. The emotional sensitivity of people with BPD results in others worrying that what they are going to say is going to be misunderstood, misconstrued, or taken to an extreme.

Bobby's parents were worried that he was going to harm himself. When he was emotionally distraught, he would run hooks through his arms. He lived at home and was in danger of dropping out of college because of too many absences. Bobby's mother would stay home from work to try to get him out of bed and get him to class. She was angry and resentful at having to do so, but when she tried to stop she felt "like a bad mother" for not helping her son and fearful that he would drop out of school and not live a successful life. Bobby and his parents had very different ideas about how people should look. They were conservative dressers, and Bobby wore baggy pants and baseball hats all the time. He wore shirts that showed his myriad scars from self-harm. Whenever his parents tried to talk with him about his appearance, there would be a fight and Bobby would dress in a way that his parents considered more outlandish and/or would cut himself. Consequently, over time, Bobby's parents stopped talking to him about anything of importance, including the fact that he was about to be kicked out of college and his goal was to go to medical school. They felt overwhelming guilt that they had "pushed" him into self-mutilating in the past and fearful that if they said anything to him about school the results would be catastrophic.

We had a family session, and I required that everyone talk about the real issues. The parents explained to Bobby that they didn't like the way he dressed and never would but that they would stop trying to make him change. However, we all agreed that they could not stop talking about school and requiring that he get up and go to class in exchange for continued housing and financial support from them. As we did this, everyone's emotions lowered and we could problem-solve things like setting a class schedule that would be conducive to Bobby getting to class. The first time that Bobby did not get up, his mother became as anxious as she had been previously. Her urge, of course, was to stay home, get him out of bed, and get him to school. She knew that having set contingencies with Bobby about when and how she would help meant that she could not stay, but her anxiety was very high. In cases like this it's important, as it is with guilt, not to give in to the urge to go back to your old behavior, which will only perpetuate the anxiety in the long run. Bobby's mother was taught the distress tolerance methods you read about in Chapter 9 and used them to get herself to work after calling out to Bobby several times. He finally dragged himself out of bed and off to classes. When he was late for class that day, his parents did not call the professor as they had in the past but required that Bobby call and repair things with the professor himself. The last I heard from him, Bobby was on his way to medical school. University was not easy for him and his parents, but as they all began to regulate emotion, Bobby turned around. Interestingly, after he and his parents began to work effectively together, Bobby walked into my office one day in khaki pants and a button-down top. I asked him what had happened, and he said that he had decided it was time that he looked like a doctor.

Assessing the Presence of True Threat

When you are looking at your anxiety and fear, ask yourself if an actual threat is present—not your perception of a threat, but a real threat. The threat can be to you or your loved one's life, health, and overall well-being. Usually it's pretty easy to figure out if the threat is toward life or health. It's threats to overall well-being that are difficult to identify. Using the skills discussed previously, try to access your wise mind and ask yourself if your intervening will be effective in the long run for the well-being of your loved one or if what it will do is make you feel better in the here and now. If there is a threat and the potential consequences are great, make the intervention. Use your fear to motivate and mobilize you to help your loved one and bring down the fear. If the threat is not real or the consequences are not helpful, approach what is making you fearful: have the conversation, communicate the limits, or don't make the intervention even if you really, really want to do so.

One of the difficulties, of course, in dealing with people whose behaviors are out of control—suicidal, self-mutilating, substance abusing—is that you can always tell yourself there is a threat to your loved one's life, health, or well-being. The potential for that harm is ever present. When possible, think of the immediacy of the threat versus the long-term potential threat. So, bailing your loved one out of jail today may decrease your fear about her health while in jail in the short term but may reinforce criminal, dysfunctional behaviors that cause more behavioral problems (and thus more fear for you in the long run).

Dealing with fear about your loved one's behaviors and trying to be wise in your responses sometimes feels like having an ax over your head. Of course, as discussed, there are no guarantees, so it is imperative that you have support for yourself in making decisions and in dealing with the emotions that are inevitable when you love someone with BPD. I'll talk about where to get that support in Chapter 13.

*D*ealing with Despair

A final emotion you may feel in your life with someone who has BPD is despair. In DBT, we often say that people with BPD must learn to deal with the overwhelming sadness of not having life work out the way they would have wished. People with BPD have amazing capacities for compassion, passion, creativity, and a wide range of emotions. Because of their hardwired sensitivity and their inability to regulate their emotions, behaviors, and relationships, their lives end up chaotic. They lose people, jobs, opportunities. Many of my clients have told me that they woke up one day and were 50 years old and just learning how to live their lives—that they had missed so much and were filled with despair. Sometimes, when people with BPD begin to improve in therapy, hopelessness and suicidal behavior will reemerge because of the grief that they feel about having "wasted their lives."

This heartbreaking response is mirrored in the family members of people with BPD. As you watch your loved one, it's impossible not to be affected by his struggles, his torment, and the often tragic consequences of his behavior. If your loved one is not getting help, hopelessness is an abyss that you can easily fall into. It is difficult to see that life can change for your loved one. You live your life thinking of what could have been. If your loved one is getting help and improving, it's difficult not to think about all the things that could have been different if help had come earlier.

The most important thing you can do is to observe and describe your sadness (see Chapter 4). Label your thoughts ("I have thoughts that she will never be able to care for herself") and your emotions ("I have feelings of sadness and loneliness that I don't have the relationship that I want with my daughter"). Balance allowing yourself to experience the emotions and letting them go so that you are not overwhelmed by them. When you experience the emotions, experience them all the way.

Letting anything go, especially emotions, is easier said than done. Start by telling yourself every time it comes up, "I am going to let go of this." Then focus your thoughts, emotions, and behaviors on something else. Use distracting or self-soothing.

Do not, however, disregard these experiences. They are important, and if you constantly push them away or suppress them, the research shows that they will return stronger and stronger. Notice them and actually lean into the emotions a little. Describe where you feel them in your body. Let the emotions rise and fall like waves. Don't try to make them bigger than they are (trust me, they will be powerful enough). Don't try to discount or deny them. Use the acceptance skills from Chapter 4 and acknowledge your emotions to yourself. If you want to work more on mindfulness, study contemplative prayer or meditation or find a mindfulness practice. Many people now go on mindfulness retreats to have a few days to practice. Mindfulness transcends religious beliefs and can be nonreligious, depending upon who is leading the practice.

Whether you discuss your sadness with your loved one depends on where she is in her ability to tolerate emotion, the state of your relationship, and the purpose of the discussion. Sometimes people with BPD want to talk about how disappointed they are with their lives. It can be very validating for them if you say that you recognize and actually experience some of the same emotions that they experience. On the other hand, some people with BPD may take that validation as your competing with them ("You're trying to say you hurt more than I do") or that they truly are hopeless and even you feel hopeless for them. Again, it's often effective to get outside support and help in communicating something as volatile as your disappointment and sadness for your loved one.

While there is a lot you can do to try to deal with emotions like guilt, fear, and despair, there's no denying that loving someone with BPD exposes you to difficult feelings and potentially dire events. In spite of your best efforts at regulating yourself and interacting effectively with your loved one and, sometimes, in spite of your loved one's best efforts, suicide and self-harm are behaviors that those who love people with BPD often have to address—the subject of the next chapter.

Understanding Self-Harm/Suicide
and Making Decisions
about Hospitalization

You just read about some of the most difficult emotions experienced by people who care deeply about a person with BPD. There is probably no subject that raises fear and despair like the specter of suicide and other self-harm. Because these are unavoidable realities in this disorder, I'm going to devote a whole chapter to the subject. First I'll try to help you understand this highly disturbing and frightening behavior. Then I'll give you the best advice I can offer, based on both research evidence and clinical experience, for dealing with your loved one's self-destructive tendencies.

*W*hat Is Going On in Self-Harm and Suicidal Behavior?

Around 75% of people with BPD attempt suicide during their lives. Unfortunately, 8–10% of them complete suicide, and the more criteria a person meets for BPD, the higher the suicide risk. As a person who loves someone with BPD, your fear that your loved one may attempt to kill herself or succeed in killing herself is firmly supported by data. Because suicidal behavior is so scary, you may doubt the decisions that you make or you may do things that you normally would not do just to make sure your loved one stays alive.

At the end of the day, the most important thing is keeping your loved one alive. If you are not sure what to do and you are afraid that one of your choices carries more risk than the other, it is important to err on the side of caution. Although I am going to give you a lot of information and recommendations for dealing with suicidal behavior and making decisions about hospitalization, always remember: you know your loved one, and if you are truly concerned that in a particular situation he may end up committing suicide, it is more important to keep him alive than anything else.

What Is the Difference between Suicidal and Self-Harm *Behaviors?*

Let's start by making sure we are clear on terms. Self-harm behaviors, or nonsuicidal self-injurious behaviors (NSSIs), are behaviors like cutting, burning, scratching, hitting, or drinking toxic substances, such as bleach. Between 60 and 80% of people with BPD, depending upon the research you read, self-harm in some way. The important point about self-harm is that there is no intent to die. Over the years, people who self-harm have erroneously been labeled as people who engage in behaviors "as a cry for help" or "for attention." Sometimes the consequence is that people do pay attention to the person who self-harms after the nonsuicidal behavior and, of course, doing so reinforces the behavior and strengthens it over time. However, as the fields of psychology and neurobiology have found out more about self-harm behaviors and their effects on physiology, we have learned that the primary reason for self-harm is emotional regulation.

For most of us it is hard to imagine, but cutting makes some people feel better. Think about a day that you had that was awful. Everything that could go wrong did go wrong. Your emotions (anger, frustration, disgust, fear, shame, guilt) increased steadily throughout the day. Then, when you finally got home at the end of the day, you did something. You went for a long run, had a glass of wine, took a warm bath, played with your pets, cooked, or cleaned. Those activities made your emotions subside, and you felt better even if you knew you had to go right back to the same situation the next day. This is what happens with people who self-harm. Often, despite their best intentions not to cut (or whatever the NSSI is that they use), their emotions build and build. When they cut, those emotions are relieved. Sometimes all they have to do is think about cutting and the emotions begin to decrease. They get relief, and their emotions are manageable again. For people who self-harm for relief, the problem for those of us who want them to stop cutting is that cutting works so well. It works quickly and effectively. Therefore, over time it is very strongly reinforcing. Like people who use drugs to manage their emotions, people who self-harm for emotional regulation struggle with "relapsing" when the going gets tough.

The misconception that self-harm is actually suicidal behavior is fed by the statistics: Ninety percent of people with BPD who self-harm do not ultimately commit suicide, yet the fact that 10% do end up dying by suicide leads some people to the erroneous conclusion that self-harm and suicide attempts are the same behavior. What we *can* conclude from these statistics is that people who self-harm are at risk for suicide.

Suicidal behaviors include thinking about suicide (suicidal ideation), planning suicide, and

> *Self-harm does not equate with suicide, but people who self-harm are at risk for suicide.*

engaging in suicide: Sometimes suicidal behaviors are a slippery slope. Many times, they start with the person with BPD **thinking about killing herself.** For many, even thinking about suicide will provide some relief from emotional distress. If the situation or emotion that is contributing to the suicidal thoughts does not resolve, behaviors can move into the planning stage. The **planning stage** is where a lot of the warning signs discussed in the next section occur. The person with BPD may buy the means to kill herself (a gun, pills, alcohol to go with the pills). She may write letters, change her will, engage in legal activities regarding her death (health care power of attorney, "do not resuscitate" orders). Planning suicide can also provide relief. People who are chronically suicidal report that planning their death helps them feel better. Although mental health practitioners look for planning, impulsive suicide attempts may not involve periods of thinking about or planning suicide. In a sense, they skip all of the steps between the event and the suicide attempt. These people are "impulsive suicide attempters," and we will discuss them later.

Suicide attempts include the actual action of killing oneself. *The important factor in suicide attempts is the intention to die.* I hear people say

"He didn't take enough pills to be dead; therefore he didn't really want to be dead." If his intent was to be dead, my response is "Thank goodness he didn't take enough pills to be dead, because he intended to die." I don't read anything into suicidal behavior. If the person wanted to be dead, it was a suicide attempt. A failed suicide attempt, but a suicide attempt nonetheless.

Warning Signs

A lot of attention is paid to knowing the warning signs of impending suicidal behavior (giving away belongings, writing suicide notes, exhibiting an increase in energy). I recommend that you know these signs even though the major suicide organizations do not necessarily agree on all of them. The ones that everyone agrees on can be found through organizations like the American Association of Suicidology or lists created by the National Institute of Mental Health. Thomas Joiner has written several books, including *Why People Die by Suicide* and *Myths about Suicide* (see the Bibliography for details), that are excellent sources for understanding suicidal behavior, although they present his theories of suicidal behavior and not necessarily research.

Long-Term Risk Factors for Suicide

- Past suicide attempts
- A family history of suicidal behavior
- Readily available methods of suicide
- Available models for suicide (highly publicized suicides)
- Marital/relationship, job, or friendship problems
- Chronic feelings of being an outsider
- Medical problems
- Physical pain
- Anxiety
- Hopelessness
- Rigidity in thinking
- Insomnia
- High agitation

Impulsive Suicidal Behavior

It's also important, if disheartening, to know that even though the majority of people do give some warning signs just prior to their suicide attempts, a study found that around 30% of people who made near-lethal suicide attempts thought about it for less than 5 minutes and did not show any signs of withdrawal, increased hopelessness, or the like. Many, many people, in fact, engage in impulsive suicidal behaviors. The only way to conceptualize their suicidal behavior is to know the things that "set them up" for suicidal behavior. Some of these factors, called *long-term risk factors*, are listed in the box. Keep in mind, however, that even these are just some of the things to pay attention to that put your loved one at higher risk for suicidal behavior. If your loved one has these risk factors, be alert to any event that he may see as bad news—losing a job, ending a relationship—because such an event may feel to your loved one like the straw that broke the camel's back. **In the event that something like this comes up, get professionals involved immediately.**

The Effects of Contagion

One of the long-term risk factors in the box on page 215 is having models for suicide. An important risk factor for suicidal behaviors is what professionals refer to as *contagion*. Although the research debates whether suicidal behaviors are really contagious, those of us who look at risk factors for suicidal behaviors pay very close attention to our suicidal clients following other suicides. In communities, when there is one suicide, others usually follow. In my hometown, one adolescent boy committed suicide by setting himself on fire. Within two weeks, four other adolescent boys had set themselves on fire.

When there is a highly publicized suicide, other suicides inevitably occur. When fashion designer Alexander McQueen committed suicide by hanging himself in his closet, five suicides by hanging in closets occurred within 2 weeks in one small area of Great Britain, McQueen's home country. Whenever there is a suicide or a death that is presumed to be suicide—even if it is later deemed to be something else—by someone who is famous, such as Kurt Cobain, Heath Ledger (whose death was proved to be accidental), or even the "Craigslist killer," Philip Markoff, many suicidal people report increases in suicidal urges. People with BPD tell me that the public suicides increase their hopelessness, anger, and doubt in their ability to create a life worth living, more so than giving them "permission" to commit suicide, as some people believe. Clients with BPD tell me that a highly publicized suicide increases the intensity and frequency of their own suicidal thoughts. Until clients stop telling me that this is true, whenever there is a public suicide, I will continue to pay very close attention to my suicidal clients.

Suicide as Solution to a Problem

Suicidal and nonsuicidal self-injurious behaviors are maladaptive problem solving. In the economic climate of 2010, people have been committing suicide because they have lost jobs or can't find jobs after they have left them. Instead of generating other ways to solve the problem of joblessness, they see suicide as the only solution. The person may think that he is a burden on his family and by dying is lifting the burden.

Often people with BPD say, "The problem is that I am suicidal." *Being suicidal is not the original problem. It is a solution to the problem.* People with BPD frequently see suicidal behavior as the only solution to their life problems and their misery. They want to end or escape from the suffering in their lives. Unfortunately, once suicide/self-harm as an option enters someone's behavioral repertoire, it is always an option. I explain this to people with BPD and their families as being similar to drinking alcohol as a solution to one's problems, for example, getting drunk after a difficult day at work. Even if the person gives up alcohol and 20 years elapse without his drinking after a hard day at work, when he has a difficult day, the first thought that pops into his mind is that he will stop on the way home and buy a six-pack of beer. *For people who have been suicidal, especially if thinking about suicide has given them some relief, when the events and emotions that have brought up suicidal thoughts in the past reappear, so will thoughts of suicide.* One thing that we do in therapy is to help people acquire many other behaviors (or solutions to their problems) to use instead of suicide. *However, it is important to understand that suicide as a solution never goes away totally.*

As mentioned above, for people with BPD, as hard as it is to believe, one problem that

> Although suicide is no way to solve life's problems and pains, it's important to know that once it has become part of your loved one's behavioral repertoire of "solutions," it will remain an option.

suicidal and self-harm behaviors solve is that they provide relief from distressing emotion. Chronically suicidal people, as well as people who self-harm, report that thinking about, planning, and attempting suicide or cutting, burning, and the like help them feel better. Katie was a high school junior who cut herself nearly every week, without the intention of killing herself. She was a straight-A student and was very perfectionistic. Katie would get very anxious about school, and that anxiety would build as the school week went on. Her ability to concentrate on her schoolwork would decline, and she would be increasingly judgmental about her schoolwork—which, of course, would increase her anxiety, which would decrease her concentration, and the cycle would continue. She would cut herself pretty deeply on her thighs, and immediately her school anxiety would decrease. After cutting, Katie would be able to concentrate on her schoolwork and perform to her own standards.

Leslie felt very lonely. She lived in a different state from her parents and had few friends. Leslie's loneliness would be worse on the weekend, and she made several suicide attempts, always on the weekend. Leslie said that she tried to kill herself so that she wouldn't feel lonely anymore (attempt at problem solving). However, she also noticed that when she made the attempts she got a "reset" on her negative emotions and started over at a less emotional place.

Negative Reinforcement: Problem Solving That Creates Its Own Problem

Research has found that there is a group of people who get relief from overwhelming emotions and feel better by even *thinking* about suicide. Stacy Shaw Welch did a study where she hooked people up to machines that measured their physiological arousal. When chronically suicidal people (people who always have some baseline suicidality) were given imaginal scenarios where they died, even accidentally or by a disease, their physiological arousal (and therefore emotional arousal) decreased. Research is still being done to figure out the physiological reasons that suicidal behavior and self-harm behavior work to regulate emotions and provide relief, but it is clear that the behaviors do work.

This phenomenon is what is called *negative reinforcement*. That means the suicidal behavior removes aversive or unpleasant emotions/situations. Think of that obnoxious buzzing, beeping, or ringing that your seat belt makes if you don't buckle it. Buckling your seat belt ends the obvious noise and reinforces seat-belt-buckling behavior. Suicidal/self-harm behaviors end the pain but function to reinforce the behavior, making it harder to get out of the person's behavioral repertoire. In the case of Welch's research, for some people, even imagining the moment of being dead helps to remove those negative feelings and thoughts.

Suicide as an Expression of Pain

Finally, suicide and self-harm behaviors can function as a way to communicate how much pain people are experiencing. As explained in Chapter 1, people who are suicidal are in an incredible amount of pain. Sometimes others mobilize around the pain, but at other times they don't. Sometimes the people in the suicidal person's environment don't "get" the pain that the person with BPD is in, either because they just don't understand it or because they have become desensitized or somewhat immune to ongoing suicidal behavior. Sometimes, as discussed in Chapter 8, the person with BPD does not have the ability to communicate accurately to others how much pain she is in. Suicidal behavior can function to show others how bad things really are for the person with BPD.

Over the years, people with BPD have developed a reputation for engaging in suicidal behaviors or self-harm as "attention seeking." They are portrayed inaccurately as making pseudo–suicide attempts, behaviors that are not really suicidal, to get others to give them attention. There are two problems with this theory. In my experience, suicidal behaviors have never begun as ways of looking for attention. People usually start suicidal behavior because they truly want relief from the tragedy and emotions of their lives.

Bill was estranged from his partner. They had been "temporarily" separated for over a year. Bill wanted reconciliation and was willing to do whatever was necessary to solve the problems in his relationship. One night, after a difficult parting with his children, who were still living with the partner, Bill went home, took a partially full bottle of sleeping pills and half a bottle of bourbon, and ended up in the emergency room. Bill's partner was called since he was still the emergency contact. He came to the emergency room and, upon seeing Bill's condition, began crying, holding Bill's hand, and promising to work on the reconciliation. After a few weeks the partner's promised behavior fizzled out. Bill was seeing his partner less and less and was hopeless again. He made another suicide attempt, and the partner came to the hospital again. Over time, the suicidal behavior increased as Bill's brain (without his awareness) began to associate suicidal behavior with changes in his partner's behavior. Bill was not just attempting suicide to get attention from his partner. His brain had learned to associate suicidal behavior with changes in his partner. So, when his emotional pain was really high, Bill had a reinforcer in place for suicidal behavior and the attention increased the likelihood of the behavior. Again, it is important to understand that that doesn't mean that Bill was intentionally engaging in suicidal behavior to "get attention" from his partner.

Sometimes suicidal behaviors are associated with attention from others—family, friends, nurses in the emergency room. The suicidal behavior may, over time, be reinforced by attention from others and

---

Potential Reinforcers of Suicidal Behavior

Things you might do that inadvertently reinforce suicidal behavior:

- Talking to your loved one more often or longer
- Being kinder or gentler
- Repairing or apologizing for your behavior when you don't usually do so
- Visiting your loved one in the hospital or ER following suicide attempts
- Changing any of your behaviors immediately following suicidal behaviors to something that your loved one would work to get (increased support, your backing off from demands that you make on her)
- Adolescents could find withdrawal of your time and attention reinforcing (as opposed to others, who would find it punishing)

Other things that can reinforce suicidal behavior:

- Getting emotional/physiological relief from the behavior
- Going to the hospital and having a "break" from stressors
- Not having to live with the demands of everyday life if they were perceived as overwhelming (getting time off from work, not having to care for home, pets, kids, partners)

may elicit helping behavior or attention. That does not mean that your loved one is "seeking attention." The difference can seem subtle but is important. If you think that the behavior is attention seeking, you may become judgmental and punitive when your loved one is suicidal. Ultimately, judgments will not help you, your loved one, or your relationship. Making judgments will make you less effective with your loved one, and you will end up being invalidating toward her.

If you are worried that you are reinforcing suicidal behavior, or doing what 12-step programs call "enabling" suicidal behavior, find a therapist who can help you identify options and change your behaviors or go to some 12-step meetings. Do not try to change the reinforcers without consultation from a professional or without the knowledge of your loved one's therapist, if she has one.

*W*hat to Do If Your Loved One Is Suicidal

There are two basic types of suicidality: chronic and acute.

Chronic suicidality is long-term suicidality. People who are chronically suicidal are often those who get relief from suicidal thoughts. They may have constant passive suicidal ideation: wishing they were dead, wishing they wouldn't wake up in the morning, not caring if they were killed in a traffic accident. Suicide is a constant in the lives of chronically suicidal people. The option is ever present, and they usually make multiple suicide attempts over the course of their lives.

Acute suicidality is a response to extreme and/or overwhelming stressors in a person's life that leads to intent to commit suicide. Acutely suicidal people are considered to be at higher risk than those who are chronically suicide. Often, people remain chronically suicidal until the stressors in their lives overwhelm them and push them into being acutely suicidal. If your loved one is basically "always" suicidal, she is chronically suicidal. It is important to note that chronically suicidal people can become acutely suicidal, so it is not effective to invalidate their chronic suicidality or act as if they will never kill themselves.

Promote Meaning and Hope

The best thing to do if your loved one is chronically suicidal is to help her create a life that does not lead to suicide. People who have relationships that are reinforcing and activities that are meaningful do not usually kill themselves. It is those who have lost the relationships and meaningful activities or who never have had them who become suicidal.

Having hope for your loved one in the absence of his hope is often helpful. It is important that you generate hope without invalidating the current experience of your loved one. So, instead of saying, "Oh, things will get better," which may force him to communicate through suicidal behaviors that they won't get better, say, "I know you don't have hope right now. It's hard to have hope, but I have hope for you. Will you let me have the hope for you?"

> *Validate the pain and hopelessness, then counteract it by generating hopeful statements.*

Communicate the Impact of Losing the Person

Another thing you can do that is helpful for chronic (and acute) suicidal behavior is to express the impact that your loved one's suicide would have on you and your family. Many times, suicidal people believe that their loved ones will be better off without them—that they are a burden on their family. As a way of showing clients the consequences of suicide for their children, we often tell them that one of the risk factors for suicide is having a family member who has completed suicide. Telling your loved one what her suicide would mean to you or writing it in a letter can be helpful. If you are doing this, be sure to use descriptive words and not euphemisms. Use the express words *suicide, kill yourself,* and *your death* and say specifically what it would mean to you. ***Do not do this if your loved one is extremely angry with you, however, because she may kill herself to show you how angry she is.***

What to Do When Your Loved One Tells You She Is Planning Suicide

If your loved one with BPD tells you, either in person or on the phone, that she is planning to kill herself, especially if she can tell you what the plan is, contact her therapist immediately. There is not a suicide specialist, no matter what type of therapy he or she does, who thinks that suicidal behavior can be treated during office hours. Most suicide attempts occur in the evenings, on the weekends, or over holidays, when therapists are not scheduled to work. If you have influence with your loved one, recommend that she find a therapist who will take after-hours calls and recommend, during a suicide crisis, that she call her therapist, get some coaching on what to do, and call you back to check in. Telling your loved one to call you back communicates concern and caring along with an expectation that she talk with the professionals. If your loved one does not have a therapist and calls you in a suicide crisis, call the local crisis clinic, mobile crisis unit (if your local mental health center or hospital has one), or, if none of those exist, call 911 ("Emergency" in other countries).

How to Respond to a Suicidal Act

If your loved one calls you and she has already done something that is suicidal, find out what she has done. If she took pills, what were the names, how many, how long ago? If she has cut, where, how deep, and is she bleeding? Is she drinking or using? If so, what has she drunk, what has she taken, how much has she drunk, or how much has she used? If she is coherent and seems not to be in danger, have her call her therapist. If she is incoherent or seems unable to do things for herself, call emergency. Give them the information that you have about what she has done. There have been a few occasions when the emergency personnel asked me to keep my client on the telephone because they did not want her to sit or lie down. I have stayed on the phone with the client to help her retain consciousness.

The Pros and Cons of Hospitalization

There is a lot of discussion about hospitalization with people who have BPD. For many years, the accepted treatment for suicidal behavior was psychiatric hospitalization. In 1993, when I began treating people with BPD, many of my clients had been hospitalized 20 to 30 times, not including the trips to the emergency room that did not result in hospitalization. If clients said they were suicidal, they were almost immediately taken to hospitals, especially if they met criteria for BPD. The common belief was that psychiatric hospitals were the only way to keep people with BPD alive. However, many of us who worked with people who were hospitalized believed that hospitals made people with BPD worse. In 1991, when I was working to help discharge patients from a state psychiatric hospital, over 80% of the patients who remained in the hospital after deinstitutionalization (a push in the 1970s and 1980s to close state hospitals and discharge people who did not need to be maintained in institutions) met criteria for BPD. Hospital social workers told stories of trying to get people with BPD ready to be discharged from the hospital only to have them jump out of buildings and ingest things like razors and glass. Anecdotally at the time, hospital staff said, "Hospitals make people with BPD worse, to the point that they can't be discharged."

In 2002, Garlow, D'Orio, and Purselle reported in the journal *Psychiatric Services* that decreasing the number of psychiatric hospital beds had not increased suicide rates as people had feared it would. Thus, moving treatment out of hospitals and into outpatient settings was not leading to more suicides. Recently, several studies have shown that hospitalization is not effective in decreasing suicide.

One of the hypotheses about why DBT is so effective at decreasing suicidal behaviors in people with BPD is that it keeps them out of the hospital. DBT therapists are not great proponents of psychiatric hospitalization, for several reasons. There are no data showing that putting people in the hospital helps them make changes in their lives outside of hospitals or that it keeps them alive. Depending upon the study you read, between 5% and 16% of all suicides are committed in inpatient psychiatric units. The highest-risk time for someone who is suicidal is immediately after being released from an inpatient unit, and 37% of males and 57% of females who commit suicide have been hospitalized. There are many ways to interpret these data, but one thing that is clear is that hospitalization does not resolve suicidal behavior. Many times therapists and family members support hospitalization because they think that the person with BPD will be discharged with suicidal behavior under control. This is not the case. Often, we hospitalize people because we are afraid that they will kill themselves if we do not hospitalize them.

So, when do you (or someone else) facilitate hospitalization for your loved one with BPD? The first instance is when her suicidal behavior is ongoing, she is very physically and emotionally perturbed (she has insomnia, her anxiety, agitation, and/or anger are very high, or she is extremely hopeless), and she cannot say that she will not kill herself. In these instances, professionals who are familiar with the research may recommend an acute (1- to 5-day) hospitalization. The purpose of the hospitalization is to get her some sleep, decrease anxiety, and, as much as possible, keep her removed from lethal means. If you think your loved one is in this state, get her help. Do not try to deal with it yourself.

The second time that you would advocate for hospitalization is if you are at the end of your rope and your loved one is acutely suicidal. Many times, suicide crises for people with BPD can last days or even weeks. During that period, many of us who care for the person with BPD are very involved in the crisis. Your loved one may be calling you for help repeatedly. You may be spending extra time with her. You may be offering all of the support you can, and naturally you begin to wear out. DBT therapists have guidelines for hospitalization, and one of them is that the system involved with the person with BPD needs a break from the suicide crisis. In other words, we will advocate for a short stay in a hospital for a person with BPD when her support system needs a break or it will burn out.

Finally, I have found that sometimes a brief (again, 1–5 days) stay in the hospital gives a person with BPD a graceful way to end the crisis. For people with BPD, especially when they are in one of the periods of unrelenting crisis (see Chapter 9), there is no end to the crisis. Ineffective decisions lead to problem consequences and more impulsive behaviors. The consequences of those behaviors lead to more impulsive behaviors. Emotions are heightened and unrelenting, leading to even more impulsive behaviors and negative consequences. There is no end in sight and no way for your loved one to stop the cycle of problem behaviors. A brief hospitalization allows the behaviors to end. Basically, going to the hospital gives your loved one a "do-over." When she is discharged, there are still the consequences of all of the impulsive behaviors to deal with, but she is out of the cycle of emotions and behaviors. This is not something I advocate often because it can reinforce "do-over" behavior, but in some instances, finding a way to end the crisis with hospitalization has been effective.

Vicky was having a difficult time with her partner. She was afraid their relationship was going to end. She had been calling her mother night after night to talk about the relationship, and finally her mother had told her that she could not tolerate hearing any more negatives about the partner and was afraid that they would not break up, leaving her with all of the negative information that Vicky had given her about the partner. Vicky had a difficult day at work and went out for a drink afterward. She had several drinks and slept with a person she met at the bar. After spending the night away from home because she was having sex with another woman, Vicky was afraid to go home and face her partner. She went back to the bar and did not go to work. This cycle went on for several days. As she realized that her job and her relationship were in serious jeopardy, she became increasingly suicidal. She began calling her mother and telling her that she was going to kill herself. However, she did not go home, did not go to work, and was living in hotels and bars. She was running out of money and did not know how to go talk with her partner or her supervisor. Finally, she was admitted to the hospital for 3 days. During the hospitalization, she got sober and began to think about how to repair relationships. Vicky lost her job because of missing so much work but managed to work out her relationship. The hospitalization gave her a way to end the problematic behaviors. When she was discharged, she had to go home to the partner and pick up the pieces of her life. During the time immediately after discharge from the hospital, she was considered at high risk for suicide and I, as her therapist, increased my contact with her to help her make decisions about managing her life and to provide support.

*H*elping Yourself

When you love someone with BPD and he or she has periods of suicidality, the stress is very high for everyone. How much you are involved really depends on how much you can tolerate. Some family members can handle extended periods of crisis, and others cannot tolerate ongoing suicidal behaviors. I am in favor of helping your loved one when (1) you are clear that it is within your own limits, (2) you are not burning out from it, (3) it is in your loved one's best interest, and (4) there are really no other options—if you don't do something, there is a high probability that the catastrophe may indeed occur. As we are going to discuss in the next chapter, living with and/or loving someone who is suicidal is difficult and scary, and I highly recommend that you find a therapist. Someone who is knowledgeable in suicide research and treatment can provide you with support and guidance in helping yourself and your loved one.

Getting Treatment and Support

In the manual for DBT, the form of therapy I use to help people with BPD, Marsha Linehan says that "therapists treating borderline personality disorder need support." I believe this is true for people who love someone with BPD as well. You need support. As discussed throughout this book, it is often hard to regulate your emotions and make wise decisions in the face of the overwhelming emotions and sometimes frightening behaviors of your loved one with BPD. Another of the core beliefs of DBT therapists is that clients "are doing the best they can." These statements were all made over 15 years ago. In more recent years, experts have stated uncategorically that the same is true of families. I believe that all of us are doing the best we can. In every moment of our lives, we are truly doing the thing that we are most capable of, the best we can do in that moment. It doesn't mean that we couldn't have chosen a wiser or a better path, but we don't say, "I am just going to mess this up intentionally right now."

It is really important to remember this belief when you are dealing with your loved one and feel the urge to say that she is deliberately ruining her life. People don't deliberately destroy their lives. They muddle through as best they can. One of the reasons that people with BPD are encouraged to get into therapy is so that they can learn more skillful ways to behave in order to experience fewer catastrophic outcomes. The same is true for people who love those with BPD. You are doing the best that you can in each moment, given your current circumstances and what you have in your arsenal of tools to deal with life and your loved one. It is important to remind yourself of this: *you are doing the best you can.* It is also important, in the heat of the moment, to remind yourself that your loved one is doing the best she can. Doing this really helps regulate emotion. However, it doesn't solve the problem that people don't have the requisite skills to do things differently. In this chapter, we are going to discuss treatment options for your loved one and resources for helping yourself.

> *It's essential to remind yourself that you're doing the best you can—and that so is the person with BPD.*

The first, most readily apparent way to help your loved one find good ways to solve her life problems is to get her into an effective therapy for BPD and/or suicidal behaviors. But this book is for you, so I want to talk about the resources you can tap for yourself first.

*R*esources That Offer Assistance and Support for You

You can feel awfully alone in trying to do your best for yourself and a person with BPD. This is particularly true because many people who qualify for a diagnosis of BPD are not in therapy. They either refuse to go to therapy or they have dropped out (or been kicked out) of therapies. Prior to the development of the evidence-based treatments described in the second half of this chapter—and, I am sorry to say, even now—people with BPD received horrendous treatment in the mental health system. Therapists, like loved ones, can fall into the abyss with people with BPD and become despairing and ineffective. It is entirely possible that your loved one has had such bad experiences in the mental health system that she refuses to be in any treatment. Don't try to force it. Therapy does not work if people are forced to go. DBT therapists will not take clients into treatment involuntarily. **If your loved one will not go to treatment, you go.**

Many DBT programs are now offering what are called "Friends and Families" groups. These groups do not require that your loved one be in DBT or any other treatment. The purpose is not to discuss your loved ones but to teach you the skills needed in emotional regulation, distress tolerance, interpersonal effectiveness, and mindfulness. These skills are helpful in dealing with your loved one but are also helpful in creating a balanced lifestyle. The groups last for 6 months and require homework and practice. They are not "therapy" but classes about learning and practicing new behaviors. Of course, family members who have been in the Friends and Families groups report that learning the skills has helped them be more effective when dealing with their loved one with BPD.

There are also two main advocacy/family support organizations that were created for family members of people with BPD. TARA (Treatment and Research Advancements, National Association for Personality Disorder) provides support and education for BPD. TARA offers family education for loved ones of people with BPD and has chapters around the country that provide the classes and other support. TARA has a very informative website and a referral center at *www.tara4bpd. org*. The National Education Alliance for Borderline Personality Disorder (NEABPD; *www.borderlinepersonalitydisorder.com*) is facilitated by researchers, therapists, and family members of people with BPD. Like TARA, NEABPD offers a course for families, called "Family Connections," a 12-week educational course at various locations across the country. Both organizations are dedicated to advancing awareness, research, and treatment of BPD while supporting loved ones.

The National Alliance for Mental Illness (NAMI; *www.nami.org*) was established in 1979 to provide support, education, and advocacy for people and families with mental illness. Originally, NAMI mostly provided programs for schizophrenia, depression, and bipolar disorder, but it now includes BPD as one of the disorders for which it provides services. NAMI has an extensive educational and support system. It offers Family to Family courses that are 12 weeks of training on behaviors (symptoms), research, decreasing caregiver burden, and increasing empathy. Family to Family is for any family member of a person with BPD, schizophrenia, bipolar disorder, depression, posttraumatic stress disorder, panic disorder, or obsessive–compulsive disorder, so it does not focus solely on the challenges of BPD. NAMI is highly visible in national, state, and local legislative movements that support treatment and treatment research.

In earlier chapters, I mentioned mindfulness as an integral part of DBT and other psychotherapy treatments. Mindfulness is a way to fully experience life and to accept each moment. Family members have found it helpful to find their own mindfulness practice. As I said earlier, mindfulness does not have to be associated with any specific religious practice. There are retreats and centers all over the country. A variety of retreats are detailed in *www.retreatfinder.com*. Jon Kabat-Zinn developed a treatment called mindfulness-based stress reduction, and he offers retreats (*www.umass.edu*). Marsha Linehan, through the Behavioral Research and Therapy Clinics at the University of Washington (*www.brtc.psych.washington.edu*) and through the Marie Institute of Behavioral Technology (*www.behavioraltech.org/marieinstitute*), offers mindfulness retreats that are predominantly designed for therapists but that family members may attend.

As discussed in Chapter 12, many people with BPD are actively suicidal, are intermittently suicidal, or have histories of suicide. However, some people with BPD never attempt suicide. *Suicide prevention* is a term for organizations that mobilize communities, hospitals, and mental health practitioners to educate families and others about the warning signs for suicide. The American Association of Suicidology (*www.suicidology.org*) provides excellent services that include helplines and certification of crisis workers for suicide. I highly recommend that you use the AAS as a resource if your loved one is suicidal.

If you, for some reason, don't want to be involved in an organization, get a therapist. Make sure the therapist has experience with BPD. I would recommend that you ask the therapist if he or she has treated people with BPD. All therapists are taught about BPD in graduate school, but there is a big difference between being educated and being experienced in treating BPD. Because you may feel naturally defensive for your loved one or yourself, pay attention to the therapist's language. Does the therapist use judgmental language when talking about your loved one? Ask questions about the therapist's theory regarding how BPD develops over time. Does the therapist blame your loved one or the people who were involved in child rearing? Ask how the therapist is going to support you. Is the therapist going to recommend that you end the relationship with your loved one? Unfortunately, BPD is a highly stigmatized disorder, and there are still therapists who believe that the best solution for family members is to terminate the relationship. Will the therapist consult with you about how to regulate your emotions and actions, or will the therapist want to delve into your childhood? There are therapists whose way of helping you in dealing with your loved one is to go through your own childhood issues. Make sure you check the training, licensing, and credentials of the therapist. Insurance will most probably not pay for you to see a therapist to help you with your loved one, but the professional support and encouragement will be worthwhile if it is affordable. The important thing is that you receive support, encouragement, and consultation, especially if your loved one with BPD is behaviorally out of control.

Finally, if you had searched the Internet for "borderline personality disorder" at the time this chapter was written, you would have found 1,220,000 entries. A search for BPD treatment would have yielded 1,320,000 results. There is a lot of misinformation about BPD and BPD treatment on the Web. You will encounter treatment groups offered by people who have no training or experience. I get phone calls from family members who are concerned because their loved ones are getting Internet therapy from people who have formed support groups or a skills group for BPD and are getting worse. There is no recourse for you or your loved one if you fall prey to unlicensed, untrained people providing "treatment." They are not accountable to any organization or bound by any ethics or laws. If you or your loved one is looking for a treatment provider or a support group and you are unsure where to look, contact one of the advocacy organizations mentioned in this chapter or in the Resources at the back of the book or consult with a mental health provider you trust. Some of the advocacy programs cannot give specific referrals, but they can help you figure out how to look. Many clients with BPD and their family members find online support groups helpful. If you are going to join one, vet the group with a professional who is familiar with BPD.

Treatments Available to the Person with BPD

Because so many of the interactions with our loved ones are emotionally charged, just making a decision about whether to approach the person with BPD and offer to intervene on his behalf or help him find professional treatment can be agonizing. On occasion, you may have to decide whether to involve professionals with or without your loved one's permission. Sometimes just thinking about confronting the person with BPD is daunting. And, as I said earlier, it's entirely possible that your loved one has already refused treatment. But if your relative is open to seeking help—or in case he becomes open at some point—you can assist by knowing what the scientific evidence says about effective therapies.

Dialectical Behavior Therapy

I practice DBT, and I recommend it most highly because it is the only treatment that demonstrates more than a 50% decrease in suicidal behaviors in the clients treated with it. Granted, we need to do much better than 50%, but DBT is constantly evolving and working to make itself more effective at treating suicidal behaviors. DBT works on the premise that people who have lives that include meaningful relationships, activities, and purpose do not attempt suicide. In other words, to be less suicidal, people have to have a life worth living. I have never met someone who said, "I have people I love and who love me, a job I enjoy, and hobbies that keep me engaged, and I want to die." People become suicidal or engage in problem behaviors because they do not believe they have love or meaning and often because they are consumed by overwhelming despair about what has happened in their lives and hopelessness about what will happen in the future. People with BPD try to escape painful emotions. DBT can help your loved one regulate emotions, experience reality as it is, repair broken relationships, create new relationships, and create meaningful activity in the service of meeting her own life goals. DBT does this by teaching new behaviors in tolerating distress, regulating emotion, practicing mindfulness, and maintaining good interpersonal relationships. DBT works on yearlong (sometimes 6-month) contracts and requires two sessions, individual therapy and group skills training, each week. DBT does offer clients telephone access to their individual therapists after hours in the hopes that your loved one will call us for coaching in crises (maybe even instead of you). In 2011, DBT therapists will begin to be certified, and you will be able to find a list of those therapists who are credentialed by Marsha Linehan and the University of Washington. To keep up with what is happening with DBT or to find a DBT therapist, go to *www.brtc.psych.washington. edu* or *www.behavioraltech.org*.

Mentalization-Based Therapy

There are other therapies being researched for treating BPD that have some promise. None of them has the impact on suicidal behaviors that

DBT has, nor do they have the research evidence that DBT has. I am going to give you a brief overview of each, designed not to educate you on the treatment but to show that there are options. Mentalization-based therapy (MBT) was originally an 18-month partial-hospitalization treatment but is now sometimes offered in a 2-year group program that alternates group and individual psychotherapy. Mentalization is described as the ability to see your emotions, thoughts, and needs and those of the people around you, to understand how emotions and needs impact your and others' actions, and to separate from them.

For example, Jane asks her husband, David, if she looks fat in an outfit. David tells her that it makes her look broad through the hips. They continue to get ready and go to the party. At the party, David thinks that Jane is avoiding him, and his feelings are hurt. On the way home from the party, they have an argument that ends in Jane drinking to the point of blacking out. Mentalization requires that David be able to look at possible explanations for Jane's behavior (he hurt her feelings; she didn't want to know what he really thought and wanted reassurance that she looked good) and that Jane be able to look at possible explanations for David's behavior (he was rushed and didn't take the time to be more gentle; he didn't know she had just bought the dress). If both David and Jane had been able to separate themselves from the event, the argument that ensued in the car going home may not have occurred. MBT posits that people with BPD do not know how to mentalize because of disrupted or problematic child rearing. MBT seeks to help people with BPD develop mentalization skills in group therapy and through interactions with an individual psychotherapist. If you think your loved one might be interested in exploring this form of therapy, organizations like TARA can steer you to providers.

Schema-Focused Therapy

Schema-focused therapy (SFT) has integrated several types of treatment (cognitive therapy, behavior therapy, object relations therapy, and mindfulness meditation). SFT views problems that people with BPD experience as stemming from problematic schemas (patterns and themes of relating to oneself and others) that developed in childhood and continue to evolve throughout life. SFT's goal is to stop people with BPD from engaging in dysfunctional behaviors and modify the problematic schemas that were developed from damaging childhood relationships. SFT uses "Limited Reparenting" and deals with the relationship between the client and the therapist, the client's life outside of therapy, and the client's childhood. SFT requires at least one session per week for 3 years. There is one randomized controlled trial (the gold standard for psychotherapy research) that measured it against transference-focused therapy but not against the standard (or usual) treatment in the community, DBT or MBT. Schema-focused therapy has a website at *www.schematherapy.com*.

Transference-Focused Psychotherapy

Transference-focused psychotherapy (TFP), like MBT, is a psychoanalytic approach. Like DBT and MBT, it is highly structured. It is based on Otto Kernberg's object relations therapy. TFP views BPD as evolving from a biological vulnerability and an environment that results in the person with BPD being unable to differentiate self from others or read social cues and developing "immature defense mechanisms" such as omnipotent control (overcontrolling others because she thinks she is being overly controlled by others), splitting (the inability to integrate "good" and "bad" in herself and others), and projection (putting her own undesirable qualities onto someone else), which result in dysfunctional behaviors, paranoia, and interpersonal fears. TFP believes that strong, unresolved negative emotions impede the ability of the person with BPD to fully separate his experiences from those of others. TFP uses the relationship with the therapist, called a *transferential relationship*, as a medium through which the person with BPD will display dysfunctional behaviors and they can be changed.

MBT, SFT, and TFP are not as prevalent as DBT and do not have the research behind them but are under development and research. The most important thing is to find a therapist who does a specialized, research-based treatment of BPD and who can demonstrate to you in some way (through credentials, test results, demonstration of supervision by experts) that he or she does the treatment *exactly* as it was researched. If you cannot find a specialist in BPD, I recommend a cognitive-behavioral therapist (again, look at credentials).

In the best case, both you and your loved one with BPD will seek (and find) support and treatment. Treatments for the disorder are being developed and tested every day. The stigma of BPD is still prevalent in our society, but in the mental health field it is fading. When I first began treating BPD, many therapists refused to give people this diagnosis because they saw it as a sentence to a horrific life and terrible mental health treatment. We didn't have effective treatments then. I was at a conference for BPD this summer, and a world leader in mental health said that the disorder is now considered "treatable" and that people want to study it. Although we have a long way to go, I considered his reflections a sign that there is hope for people with BPD and their loved ones. Use the Resources section that follows to find help now and to keep abreast of changes in the treatment of BPD.

Resources

*T*herapies That Treat Borderline Personality Disorder

Dialectical Behavior Therapy

Behavioral Research and Therapy Clinics
Department of Psychology
University of Washington
3935 University Way NE
Seattle, WA 98195
Phone: 206-543-BRTC (206-543-2782)
Website: *http://blogs.uw.edu/brtc/*

Mentalization-Based Therapy[1]

Anthony Bateman
Halliwick Day Unit
St. Ann's Hospital
St. Ann's Road
London N15 3TH, England
Phone: 020 8442 6093
Fax: 020 8442 6545
E-mail: *anthony@abate.org.uk*

Peter Fonagy
Room 541
Psychoanalysis Unit
1–19 Torrington Place

---

[1]Does not have a specific website but can be reached through the treatment developers' labs.

London WC1E 7HB, England
Phone: 020 7679 1943
Fax: 020 7916 8502
E-mail: *p.fonagy@ucl.ac.uk*

Schema-Focused Therapy

Schema Therapy Institute
561 10th Avenue, Suite 43D
New York, NY 10036
Phone: 212-594-9494, x200
Fax: 212-837-2741
E-mail: *institute@schematherapy.com*
Website: *www.schematherapy.com*

Transference-Focused Psychotherapy

New York Presbyterian Hospital—Westchester Division
21 Bloomingdale Road
White Plains, NY 10605
E-mail: *info@borderlinedisorders.com*
Website: *www.borderlinedisorders.com*

*O*rganizations

United States

American Association of Suicidology
5221 Wisconsin Avenue NW
Washington, DC 20015
Phone: 202-237-2280
Fax: 202-237-2282
National Suicide Prevention Lifeline, 1-800-273-TALK
Website: *www.suicidology.org*

Behavioral Research and Therapy Clinics
Department of Psychology
University of Washington
3935 University Way NE
Seattle, WA 98195
Phone: 206-543-BRTC (206-543-2782)
Website: *https://blogs.uw.edu/brtc/*

Behavioral Tech, LLC/The Linehan Institute
4746 11th Avenue NE, Suite 102
Seattle, WA 98105
Phone: 206-675-8588
Fax: 206-675-8590
Websites: *www.behavioraltech.org, www.linehaninstitute.org*

National Alliance on Mental Illness
3803 North Fairfax Drive, Suite 100
Arlington, VA 22203
Phone: 703-524-7600
Fax: 703-524-9094
Member Services: 888-999-NAMI (6264)
Website: *www.nami.org*

National Education Alliance for Borderline Personality Disorder
P.O. Box 974
Rye, NY 10580
E-mail: *info@borderlinepersonalitydisorder.com*
Website: *www.borderlinepersonalitydisorder.com*

Treatment Implementation Collaborative, LLC
6327 46th Avenue SW
Seattle, WA 98136
Phone: 206-251-5134
Website: *www.ticllc.org*

Treatment and Research Advancements, National Association for Personality Disorder
23 Greene Street
New York, NY 10013
Phone: 212-966-6514
Website: *www.tara4bpd.org*

Canada

Canadian Mental Health Association
National Office
1110-151 Slater Street
Ottawa, ON K1P 5H3, Canada
Phone: 613-745-7750
Fax: 613-745-5522
General Inquiries: *info@cmha.ca*
Website: *www.cmha.ca*

Health Canada
Address Locator 0900C2
Ottawa, ON K1A 0K9, Canada
Phone: 613-957-2991 or 866-225-0709
Fax: 613-941-5366
Teletypewriter: 800-267-1245 (Health Canada)
General Inquiries: *Info@hc-sc.gc.ca*
Website: *www.hc-sc.gc.ca*

United Kingdom

BPD World
Website: *www.bpdworld.org*

Carers UK
Phone: 020 7378 4999
Carers line: 0808 808 7777
Website: *www.carersuk.org*

Carers Northern Ireland
Phone: 028 9043 9843
Website: *www.carersni.org*

Carers Scotland
Phone: 0141 445 3070
Website: *www.carerscotland.org*

Carers Wales
Phone: 029 2081 1370
Website: *www.carerswales.org*

Carers and Users Support Enterprise
Phone: 028 90 650 650 or 0845 60 30 29 1 (Helpline)
Website: *www.cause.org.uk*

Mental Health Foundation
Phone: 08457 90 90 90
General Inquiries: *jo@samaritans.org*
Website: *www.mentalhealth.org.uk*

Mental Health Foundation Scotland
Phone: 0141 572 0125
General Inquiries: *scotland@mhf.org.uk*
Website: *www.mentalhealth.org.uk/about-us/scotland/*

Mind
Information Line: 020 8519 2122
E-mail: *contact@mind.org.uk*
Website: *www.mind.org.uk*

National Collaborating Centre for Mental Health
Phone: 0207 977 6677
General Inquiries: *info@nccmh.org.uk*
Website: *www.nccmh.org.uk*

National Self Harm Network
General Inquiries: *info@nshn.co.uk*
Website: *www.nshn.co.uk*

Northern Ireland Association for Mental Health
Phone: 028 9032 8474
Website: *www.niamhwellbeing.org*

Scottish Association for Mental Health
Phone: 0141 530 1000
General Inquiries: *enquire@samh.org.uk*
Website: *www.samh.org.uk*

New Zealand

Mental Health Foundation of New Zealand
Website: *www.mentalhealth.org.nz*

Supporting Families in Mental Illness in New Zealand
Website: *www.supportingfamiliesnz.org.nz*

Australia

Behavioural Tech
Website: *www.behavioraltech.org*
Phone: 1206 675 8588

BPD Central
www.bpdcentral.com

Carers ACT
Phone: 6296 9900
Website: *www.carersact.asn.au*

Facing the Facts
www.bpdfamily.com

Mental Health Foundation
Phone: 6282 6658
General Inquiries: *info@mhfa.org.au*
Website: *www.mhf.org.au*

SANE Australia
Phone: 3 9682 5933
General Inquiries: *info@sane.org*
Website: *www.sane.org*

$\mathcal{B}$ooks

Chapman, A., & Gratz, K. (2007). *The borderline personality disorder survival guide: Everything you need to know about living with BPD.* Oakland, CA: New Harbinger.

Fruzzetti, A. E. (2006). *The high conflict couples: A dialectal behavior therapy guide to finding peace, intimacy and validation.* Oakland, CA: New Harbinger.

Hall, K., & Cook, M. (2011). *The power of validation: Arming your child against bullying, peer pressure, addiction, self-harm and out-of-control emotions.* Oakland, CA: New Harbinger.

Hoffman, P. D., & Steiner-Grossman, P. (2008). *Borderline Personality Disorder: Meeting the challenges to successful treatment.* Philadelphia, PA: Haworth Press.

Hollander, M. (2008). *Helping teens who cut: Understanding and ending self-injury.* New York: Guilford Press.

Koerner, K. (2012). *Doing dialectical behavior therapy: A practical guide.* New York: Guilford Press.

Linehan, M. M. (1993). *Cognitive-behavioral treatment of borderline personality disorder.* New York: Guilford Press.

Linehan, M. M. (1993). *Skills training manual for borderline personality disorder.* New York: Guilford Press.

Miller, A. L., Rathus, J. H., & Linehan, M. M. (2007). *Dialectical behavior therapy for suicidal adolescents.* New York: Guilford Press.

Porr, V. (2010). *Overcoming borderline personality disorder: A family guide for healing and change.* New York: Oxford University Press.

Pryor, K. (2002). *Don't shoot the dog!: The new art of teaching and training* (3rd ed.). Dorking, UK: Interpet Publishing.

Van Gelder, K. (2010). *The Buddha and the borderline: My recovery from borderline personality disorder through dialectal behavior therapy, Buddhism and online dating.* Oakland, CA: New Harbinger.

$\mathcal{D}$ VDs

From Guilford Publications

Linehan, M. M. (2006). *Treating Borderline Personality Disorder: The Dialectical Approach.* New York: Guilford Press.

Linehan, M. M. (2006). *Understanding Borderline Personality Disorder: The Dialectical Approach.* New York: Guilford Press.

From Behavioral Tech

Chaos to Freedom (four videos on crisis skills, radical acceptance, and mindfulness) (2003). Seattle, WA: Behavioral Tech.

DBT at a Glance: An Introduction to Dialectical Behavior Therapy (2009). Seattle, WA: Behavioral Tech.

Opposite Action: An Adaptation from the Deaf Perspective (2006). Seattle, WA: Behavioral Tech.

Opposite Action: Changing Emotions You Want to Change (2000). Seattle, WA: Behavioral Tech.

Practicing Radical Acceptance: An Adaptation from the Deaf Perspective (2007). Seattle, WA: Behavioral Tech.

Bibliography

American Psychiatric Association. (2000). *Diagnostic and statistical manual of mental disorders* (4th ed., text rev.). Washington, DC: Author.

Bateman, A., & Fonagy, P. (2004). *Psychotherapy for borderline personality disorder: Mentalisation based treatment.* Oxford, UK: Oxford University Press.

Garlow, S., D'Orio, B., & Purselle, D. (2002). The relationship of restrictions on state hospitalizations and suicides among emergency psychiatric patients. *Psychiatric Services, 53,* 1297–1300.

Giesen-Bloo, J., van Dyck, R., Spinhoven, P., van Tilburg, W., Dirksen, C., van Asselt, T., et al. (2006). Outpatient psychotherapy for borderline personality disorder: A randomized trial of schema-focused therapy versus transference-focused therapy. *Archives of General Psychiatry, 63*(6), 649–658.

Gunderson, J. G., & Hoffman, P. D. (2005). *Understanding and treating borderline personality disorder: A guide for professionals and families.* Washington, DC: American Psychiatric Press.

Joiner, T. E. (2005). *Why people die by suicide.* Cambridge, MA: Harvard University Press.

Joiner, T. E. (2010). *Myths about suicide.* Cambridge, MA: Harvard University Press.

Linehan, M. M. (1993). *Cognitive-behavioral treatment of borderline personality disorder.* New York: Guilford Press.

Linehan, M. M. (1993). *Skills training manual for borderline personality disorder.* New York: Guilford Press.

Linehan, M. M. (1997). Validation and psychotherapy. In A. C. Bohart & L. S. Greenberg (Eds.), *Empathy reconsidered: New directions in psychotherapy.* Washington, DC: American Psychological Association.

Linehan, M. M. (2001). *Opposite action: Changing the emotions you want to change* (dialectical behavior therapy skills training video). Seattle, WA: Behavioral Tech, LLC.

Miller, A. L., Rathus, J. H., & Linehan, M. M. (2007). *Dialectical behavior therapy for suicidal adolescents.* New York: Guilford Press.

Pryor, K. (2002). *Don't shoot the dog!: The new art of teaching and training* (3rd ed.). Dorking, UK: Interpet Publishing.

Swann, W. B., Jr., & Read, S. J. (1981). Self-verification processes: How we sustain our self-conceptions. *Journal of Experimental Social Psychology, 17,* 351–372.

Thomas, A., & Chess, S. (1977). *Temperament and development.* New York: Brunner/Mazel.

Welch, S. S., Linehan, M. M., Sylvers, P., Chittams, J., & Rizvi, S. L. (2008). Emotional responses to self-injury imagery among adults with borderline personality disorder. *Journal of Consulting and Clinical Psychology, 76,* 45–51.

Yeomans, F. E., Clarkin, J. F., & Kernberg, O. F. (2002). *A primer of transference-focused psychotherapy for the borderline patient.* Northvale, NJ: Jason Aronson.

Index

About the Author

Shari Y. Manning, PhD, is a clinician in private practice and the former President/CEO of Behavioral Tech and Behavioral Tech Research, the organizations founded by Marsha M. Linehan to provide training in dialectical behavior therapy. Dr. Manning has focused on the treatment of people with borderline personality disorder since 1993. She lives in Columbia, South Carolina.